HOW CONNECTIONS HEAL

How Connections Heal

Stories from Relational–Cultural Therapy

Edited by
MAUREEN WALKER
WENDY B. ROSEN

Foreword by Jean Baker Miller

THE GUILFORD PRESS
New York   London

© 2004 The Guilford Press
A Division of Guilford Publications, Inc.
72 Spring Street, New York, NY 10012
www.guilford.com

Printed in the United States of America

This book is printed on acid-free paper.

Last digit is print number: 9 8 7 6 5 4 3 2 1

Library of Congress Cataloging-in-Publication Data

How connections heal : stories from relational–cultural therapy / edited
by Maureen Walker, Wendy B. Rosen.
    p. cm.
Includes bibliographical references and index.
  ISBN 1-59385-033-6 (hardcover) — ISBN 1-59385-032-8 (pbk.)
  1. Eclectic psychotherapy. 2. Cultural psychiatry. 3.
Psychotherapy—Cross-cultural studies. 4. Psychodynamic psychotherapy.
I. Walker, Maureen. II. Rosen, Wendy B.
  RC554.H69 2004
  616.89′14—dc22

                                                2003026346

About the Editors

Maureen Walker, PhD, is a licensed psychologist with an independent practice in psychotherapy and multicultural consultation in Cambridge, Massachusetts. She is a member of the faculty and the director of program development at the Jean Baker Miller Training Institute of the Stone Center at Wellesley College. Dr. Walker is a coeditor of *The Complexity of Connection* (2004, Guilford Press) and has authored several papers in the Stone Center's Works in Progress Series. She is also the associate director of MBA Support Services at Harvard Business School.

Wendy B. Rosen, PhD, is a licensed clinical social worker with a full-time private practice in Cambridge, Massachusetts. She is on the faculty of the Jean Baker Miller Training Institute and is on the attending staff of McLean Hospital in Belmont, Massachusetts. Dr. Rosen has taught for many years as a member of the adjunct faculty at Smith College School for Social Work. In 1999, she received the Massachusetts National Association of Social Workers' award for Greatest Contribution to Social Work Practice. She has also presented numerous papers and has authored and coauthored a number of published articles.

Contributors

Roseann Adams, MSW, LCSW, Illinois Department of Children and Family Services and St. James Cathedral Counseling Center, Chicago, Illinois

Dana L. Comstock, PhD, Department of Counseling, St. Mary's University, San Antonio, Texas

Nikki Fedele, PhD, Jean Baker Miller Training Institute, Wellesley College, Wellesley, Massachusetts; Brigham and Women's Hospital, Harvard Medical School, Boston, Massachusetts; private practice, Wayland, Massachusetts

Linda M. Hartling, PhD, Jean Baker Miller Training Institute, Wellesley College, Wellesley, Massachusetts

Yvonne M. Jenkins, PhD, University Counseling Services, Boston College, Boston, Massachusetts; Jean Baker Miller Training Institute, Wellesley College, Wellesley, Massachusetts; private practice, Brookline, Massachusetts

Judith V. Jordan, PhD, Jean Baker Miller Training Institute, Wellesley College, Wellesley, Massachusetts; Department of Psychiatry, Harvard Medical School, Boston, Massachusetts

Alice C. Lawler, PhD, private practice, Austin, Texas

Wendy B. Rosen, PhD, Jean Baker Miller Training Institute, Wellesley College, Wellesley, Massachusetts; McLean Hospital, Belmont, Massachusetts; private practice, Cambridge, Massachusetts

Karen Skerrett, PhD, Chicago Center for Family Health and private practice, Chicago, Illinois

Elizabeth Sparks, PhD, Department of Counseling Psychology, Boston College, Boston, Massachusetts; Jean Baker Miller Training Institute, Wellesley College, Wellesley, Massachusetts

Maureen Walker, PhD, Jean Baker Miller Training Institute, Wellesley College, Wellesley, Massachusetts; private practice, Cambridge, Massachusetts

Cynthia Walls, MA, LCSW, St. James Cathedral Counseling Center and private practice, Chicago, Illinois

Foreword

In the past, the therapeutic relationship was seen as the backdrop for the real work of therapy: that is, the interpretations, reconstructions, confrontations, reinforcements, and the like. We now see it as *the* work of therapy. Those forces that keep the patient out of connection are the forces that keep her or him from growing and thriving in life; they will occur in therapy, and in that safe context the person can begin to change them. At times, various specific techniques may be of great help, but their implementation also must rest on a productive relationship. Originally referred to as self-in-relation theory, then relational theory, and now relational–cultural theory, our name has evolved with our concepts.

"But what do you actually do differently in therapy? What's culture got to do with it?" Ever since we began talking about relational–cultural theory, people have asked these questions. This book is an attempt at an answer. It focuses on the day-to-day work of therapy and also includes a sampling of applications of the theory in larger institutions.

Culture has everything to do with psychological growth and development. The most basic assumption of relational–cultural theory is that people thrive in growth-fostering relationships in therapy, as in life. A culture that does not provide a growth-fostering impetus for everyone sets in motion forces that can end in psychological problems—and the therapeutic relationship, itself, reflects the surrounding culture in both obvious and subtle ways.

The central question becomes: What will lead to a growthful connection that is based in ever-increasing truthfulness and authenticity? The values implicit in this question guide all of psychological development as well as all therapy. The inverse question is: What interferes with the growth of relationship? The chapters in this book address these questions. While people may come to therapy at various times in their lives for various reasons, and therapy may take various forms, building the relationship constitutes the essential healing ingredient.

Trying to talk about therapy is elusive because it means trying to talk about a process in motion, not a fixed, static entity. It means talking about "movement in relationship." Therapy involves a flow between two or more people in which each (or all) tries to represent her or his experience as it is occurring—and as it is modified in the moment by the very experience each is having, because of what the other person(s) is saying, doing, feeling. This interplay is the essence of connection in therapy, as in life. Unfortunately, our culture does not provide us with good language to describe it.

Although the contributors to this volume do not yet create this desired language, they do approach this need by describing their part in the relationship more fully rather than talking more "objectively" about the patient. Of course, the focus is always on the patient's needs, but the therapist is inevitably *in* the interchange. She or he has the responsibility to make the interchange growthful for the patient, and she or he is always a participant in the relationship that will bring about that growth. Thus, the therapists here are trying to describe "the space between": not one person or the other, but the dynamic interchange between them that is the heart of therapy. For this reason many of the chapters may seem to focus unduly on the therapists. This is certainly not because these therapists have more problems than others. It is because they are willing to examine their part in the interplay more thoroughly than we typically encounter in clinical presentations. Whatever the patient's problem, it is the therapist's contribution to "the space between" that will make the difference. It is not a question of the therapist's occasional lapse into some unanalyzed bit of countertransference but the multifaceted, ever-changing "feeling-thoughts" that arise throughout the interchange and how well they will foster the growth of connection.

The therapist's task is to find the ways to keep the relationship moving toward a deepening connection. Only as the connection deepens can patients discover the nature of their particular strategies of disconnection and find the courage to confront their deepest fears or terrors. Only then can patients begin to risk feeling and acting in a new way. Only as the connection deepens can they find the disconnected parts of self. As they become more connected, they become more themselves and also find new possibilities.

When therapists truthfully examine the forces that interfere with connection in themselves and others, they often find that these forces reflect the patterns of our culture—a culture that has taught us all many ways of denying each other the fullness and richness of the connection we need for all of living. Thus, therapy is not only about the specific forms of disconnection each person has devised but the underlying societal forces that deprive and hurt many families. As families suffer harm, they develop protective forms of disconnection that scar their children. In our theory, the word *culture* connotes not only the attempt to encompass cultural differences among us but also the study of the effects of a dominant culture with which we all must contend in one way or another and within which we learn the disconnections that create our problems—and that enter into the therapy room, itself, the very setting of our attempts at healing.

In the final section of this book, the contributors apply this theory to institutional settings, where they find similar but not identical issues. The questions here also include: (1) What will lead to better connection? and (2) What are the factors interfering with connection? The contributors discover that deepening connection leads to increased effectiveness within the institution as well as growth of the individuals involved.

This book offers original pieces illustrating how therapists are currently using relational–cultural theory in clinical work as well as examples of applying the theory in larger settings. As noted above, as various practitioners apply it, relational–cultural theory evolves into a fuller, richer theory. We are convinced that it opens new vistas in therapeutic practice, and, as we grandiosely claim, we believe it offers a guide to changing the world.

JEAN BAKER MILLER, MD

Contents

Part I

An Introduction to Relational–Cultural Theory and Practice

1

How Relationships Heal

MAUREEN WALKER

As other perceptions arise . . . . the total vision of human
possibilities enlarges and is transformed.
—JEAN BAKER MILLER (1976, p. 1)

Telling a story about human possibilities is necessarily a complex
task. As it has been told through the traditional frameworks of Western
psychology, the story of human development has been both limited and
limiting. The theoretical models of Western psychology represent varia-
tions on a culture-bound story: a story marked by efforts to appear scien-
tifically objective or "neutral" (Jordan, 2001). Yet the theories typically derive from a position of cultural dominance, and so certain omissions and
distortions seem all but inevitable (Miller, 1976). To the extent that any
psychological theory ignores the sociopolitical realities of the culture in
which it arises, it can render only a fragmented interpretation of human
experience. Indeed, it was such fragmented interpretation that led Miller
(1984) to assert that certain tenets of traditional psychology, including the
notion of "self," do not seem to fit the experience of women. Miller and
others (Broverman, Broverman, Clarkson, Rosencrantz, & Vogel, 1970;
Gilligan, 1982; Stiver, 1991a) observed a direct relationship between male
gender privilege and attributions of psychological health; likewise, they
noted correspondences between female gender subordination and attributions of psychological and maturational deficiencies. These observations suggest that attempting to understand human development without
regard to the context in which it is experienced leads to distorted percep-

tions not only of the socially subordinated but of the socially privileged as well.

In light of these observations, scholars from both academic and clinical traditions began to question the integrity of psychological theories abstracted from social context, as well as the efficacy of their derivative treatment models. Accordingly, the impetus for the Jean Baker Miller relational–cultural model came from evidence that women were being misunderstood and misrepresented by prevailing psychodynamic models (Jordan, 2001). When autonomy, separation, and independence are the prevailing standards of mature psychological functioning, women by most measures are judged deficient. Rather than accept these representations as truth, Miller (1976), the group gathered around her, and other feminist theorists began to critique psychodynamic models and treatment modalities (Gilligan, 1982; Jordan, Kaplan, Miller, Stiver, & Surrey, 1991). More to the point, the founding scholars of the Jean Baker Miller relational–cultural model responded by examining the experience of their women clients.

A central tenet of the relational–cultural model is that people grow through action in relationship with others. As Jordan (2001) describes it, this model is built on an understanding of people that emphasizes a primary movement toward, and yearning for, connection with others throughout the lifespan (p. 95). In the popular imagination, connection is often exclusively associated with interpersonal ease and comfort. However, there is an important linkage between connection and what Miller (1976) has termed "good conflict." One of the founding concepts of the model is that connection inevitably includes conflict. In her seminal text, *Toward a New Psychology of Women*, Miller discusses conflict as the source of all growth and "an absolute necessity if one is to be alive" (p. 125). In both theory and in practice, the model necessarily concerns itself with questions of privilege and power. As Miller explains, conflict is a natural outgrowth of engagement with difference, including inequal status in relationship. By elucidating differences such as status inequalities, the relational–cultural model positions cultural context and the associated power dynamics as central issues in psychological functioning. The evolution of the model, from self-in-relation theory to relational–cultural theory, reflects an elaborated understanding of connection from a primarily interpersonal encounter to a complex, pluralistic process with profound implications for psychological and sociopolitical well-being.

In theory, this evolution reflects the active inclusion of voices representing the diversity of experience from the margins as well as the center in patriarchal culture. Although the founding scholars began by listening to their own and their clients' voices to better understand women's experiences, they recognized the inherent limitations of generalizing from a small group of racially and economically privileged, primarily heterosexual women to the lived experience of all women in North American culture (Kaplan, 1991). The scholars turned to writings and critiques from women and men representing a range of cultural and political backgrounds (Kaplan, 1991). Most importantly, rather than adopt an "add-on" approach, the founding scholars invited new voices into the center of the theory's development, thereby opening the process to transformational possibilities (Jordan & Hartling, 2002). The lesbian theory group and the multicultural theory group were formed, and both have contributed to a more nuanced understanding and rearticulation of key relational–cultural concepts. In this regard, the process of theory development has been a relationally emergent, evolving experience marked by early recognition that there exists not *one* psychology of women but many (Jordan & Hartling, p. 55). Furthermore, although the theory was initially developed as an attempt to understand women's development, there is increasing recognition that the core concepts illuminate processes necessary for human development (Jordan, 2002, p. 234; Miller, 1976). To paraphrase bell hooks (1984), by listening to the voices at the margins of patriarchal culture, the model can envision new alternatives for the center. Indeed, the process of theory development has remained consistent with Miller's original intent: to liberate humankind's view of itself from the limiting distortions of exclusionary bias, thereby enlarging the vision of human possibility.

COMPARISONS ACROSS "RELATIONAL" MODELS

The relational–cultural model is one among many theories of development that brings a focus on connection. Indeed, over the past several years, more than a few theories of psychological functioning have been described as relational models. In a comprehensive review of current developments in feminist psychology, infancy research, and relational psychoanalysis, Spencer (2000) identified areas of convergence and divergence among these theories, with particular emphasis on their embedded assumptions about mental health and distress, emotional healing, and maturation. Likewise, Jordan (2002) has provided succinct explanations of the distinct viewpoints and contributions of the various frameworks. In many such models, the language of connection belies a philosophical commitment to the primary of drive satisfaction in service of the separate self. Although many of the models are described as relational, they equate psychological health with the development and maintenance of a cohesive self; conversely, self-fragmentation is viewed as the primary source of psychological distress. Citing the Kohutian model as a case in point, Jordan (2002, pp. 233–234) draws a distinction between relationship with a *self-*

object, which is under the fantasized control of the individual, and relationship with a *person* who has his or her own subjectivity. To a greater or lesser degree, the goal in many of these models is individual internalization of the functions of relationship in order to become self-sustaining. It would seem, then, that the implicit goal of development is to outgrow the need for relationship. Jordan (2002, p. 234) also notes the primacy of intrapsychic structure in the two-person psychologies that grew out of the Kohutian model. Indeed in each of these, the analytic tradition of interpretation is viewed as the path to healing; the therapeutic relationship itself is at best facilitative, providing a context that maximizes the potency of the interpretation. Although these psychologies represent a clear shift from the more skeptical view of relationship as a potentially impinging stimulus that thwarts psychological development (Freud, 1955), they remain distinct from models that posit the primacy of relationship. As long as the utilitarian value of relationship is emphasized, relationship becomes yet another resource or commodity that must be acquired or mastered if the person is to enjoy optimal health. This focus on *having* or *possessing* relationship contrasts sharply with Miller's (1988) formulations about *being in* or *action in* relationship.

In relational–cultural theory, relationship is both the process and the goal of human development (Miller, 1976; Miller & Stiver, 1997). Rather than defining psychological health as movement toward increased autonomy, relational–cultural theory identifies increasing levels of complexity, fluidity, choice, and articulation within human relationship as markers of developmental maturity (Jordan et al., 1991). Psychological development is seen as taking place in and through increasingly complex relationships, and psychological health is viewed as a function of participation in relationship, in which mutually empowering connections occur (Jordan, Surrey, & Kaplan, 1991). Unlike traditional models that emphasize intrapsychic fragmentation as the cause of mental distress, relational–cultural theory views chronic disconnection as the primary source of human suffering, resulting in paralyzing psychological isolation and impaired relational functioning. Moreover, such disconnections are exacerbated by patterned and protracted abuses of power in relationship, whether the relational context is interpersonal, familial, or institutional–cultural—or, in many instances, some combination of the three.

WHAT HAPPENS IN RELATIONAL–CULTURAL THERAPY?

The purpose of this text is to illuminate the processes in relational–cultural therapy that facilitate growthful change. If the primary cause of human suffering is chronic disconnection, how can the therapeutic relationship increase capacity for resilience and empower movement toward connection? Each of the cases included in this book provides an up-close view of the therapeutic relationship, thus allowing the reader to see the theory "at work." Unlike many theories and training models that emphasize acquisition of specific tools and techniques, relational–cultural work represents a *worldview* or *philosophical approach* to healing and human development. As such, there are no "stand alone" techniques that capture the essence of relational–cultural practice. Instead, the relational–cultural practitioner works from a set of grounding values and foundational concepts that inform therapeutic decision making on a case-by-case—or more accurately, on a relationship-by-relationship—basis.

The core foundational ideas developed by the founding scholars of the relational–cultural model include the following (Jordan et al., 1991):

- Relational differentiation and elaboration, rather than separation, characterize growth.
- Mutuality and shared power are markers of mature functioning.
- Mutual empathy is an essential process in effective therapies.
- Therapeutic authenticity is necessary for the development of mutual empathy.

Because we believe that therapist authenticity and mutual empathy are essential components of effective therapy, the authors of the chapters that follow offer an inside view of their own cognitive–affective experiences in relationship with a single client, with a group or family, or with a community of persons in an institutional–organizational setting. The narratives themselves are thickly textured, revealing not only moments of intimacy, clarity, and courage, but also the patterns of disconnection, ambivalence, and uncertainty in the relationship. These candid presentations provide poignant illustrations of Miller's (1976) assertions regarding the inevitability and the usefulness of acute conflict as a source of growthful change.

Each author is an experienced clinician–educator who is committed to the values and understandings of relational–cultural theory and is contributing her work to illustrate how those values guide her decision making and translate into therapeutic action. In their case narratives, the authors also describe the presenting concerns in relation to the sociocultural variables that affect the client's, as well as their own, experience of the relationship. These variables include, but are not limited to, race/ ethnicity, gender, socioeconomic status, sexual orientation, class concerns, and health status. In addition to highlighting her decision processes, each contributor has also examined her participation in the processes of connection and the strategies of disconnection at critical junctures in the relationship. Each of the following narratives illustrates the author's attempt to facilitate processes of empathy, authenticity, and mutuality; indeed, at the base of each relationship is a commitment to these core relational practices. Also implicit to each narrative are themes of power and empowerment, movement and resilience. Although the behavioral translations of these concepts necessarily vary across relationships, embedded in each are unitive understandings about the value of good connection, the importance of conflict, the evolution of relational boundaries, and movement through vulnerability to shared power. The next section offers an orientation to our understandings of these concepts.

CONCEPTS, VALUES, AND LANGUAGE OF RELATIONAL–CULTURAL THEORY

The language of relational–cultural theory is intentionally simple. In an effort to demystify and democratize the therapeutic process, Miller and her group adopted language accessible to a larger public—a public that includes, but is not limited to, graduate-level professionals. However, the simplicity of the language belies the complexity of the work. Because the language is simple, it has, at times, lent itself to simplistic interpretation. Moreover, as with any model, terms originally intended as critical signifiers may devolve into a form of coded speech. With these evolutionary sensitivities in mind, the contributing authors have presented therapeutic relationships that provide a venue for reexamining, rearticulating, and, in some instances, reformulating foundational concepts of relational–cultural theory. As Jordan and Hartling (2002) suggest, the credibility of a theoretical model rests on the continual evaluation of its underlying assumptions in light of emergent experience.

Anyone familiar with relational–cultural practice recognizes the centrality of *connection* to psychological development. Hence, there is no better place to start than with the word connection itself. Its use within relational–cultural theory differs somewhat from its current, common usage.

Defining Connection

The word *connection* has become popular in recent years, due, in large measure, to the number of trade and self-help publications that promote relationship as a source of well-being. In conventional usage, the term is used to describe encounters characterized by interpersonal harmony, warm support, and pleasant feelings. The term may also connote a relationship among people with similar interests and inclinations, or with someone who can facilitate movement toward some desired goal. These qualities may, in fact, describe important aspects of connection; however, they do not include other critical dimensions of the process. Miller (1988; Miller & Stiver, 1997) has consistently distinguished these kinds of encounters from what she terms "growth-fostering" connection. In the relational–cultural model, connection is both *encounter* and *active process*, and its fundamental quality is *respect*. This conception of respect is akin to the concept of unconditional positive regard emphasized in person-centered models. In relational–cultural theory, however, there is the additional connotation of bidirectionality. Respect is not simply a gift bestowed upon clients by therapists. It is enabled by therapists' openness to witnessing clients' and their own complexity. To experience connection is to participate in a relationship that invites exposure, curiosity, and openness to possibility. Simply put, connection provides safety from contempt and humiliation; however, it does not promise comfort. Indeed, connection may be— and often is—a portal to increased conflict, because safety in relationship allows important differences to surface. How those differences are treated is a telling indicator of the quality of connection—that is, the extent to which an encounter embodies or engenders an increased sense of worth, clarity, zest, and desire for more relationship. To paraphrase Miller (1976), connection involves the respectful negotiation of difference that facilitates growth and the emergence of something new. In each of the cases that follows, the reader is invited to track the development of processes that facilitate movement in relationship, growth in connection. Those processes—empathy, authenticity, and mutuality—are defined later in this chapter.

The Relational Paradox

The central guide to the therapist's work is the *relational paradox* (Miller & Stiver, 1997), also called the paradox of disconnection or connection. A common response to the chronic absence of safety and respect in relationship is to resort to *strategies of disconnection*. These are ways of withdrawing from relationship for protection. They often retain an appearance of connection while lacking its substance. Miller and Stiver (1997) maintain that strategies of disconnection represent perceptions of "safe" alternatives in the face of repeated experiences of neglect, humiliation, and violation. The paradox is that these strategies, which may or may not be held in conscious awareness, mask both the *longing for* and the *terror of* connection. If the therapy is to be productive, the therapist must remain empathic as both sides of the paradox emerge in the therapist–client relationship (Miller & Stiver, 1995, 1997). If instead the therapist disconnects in reaction to this paradox, the likely result is an impasse (Stiver, 1992). Under conditions of chronic abuse and violation, a person may become more adept at behaving "as if" he or she is in connection while not actually being "present to" or active in the relationship (Stiver, 1990). When the dominant culture itself is the agent of disconnection (Jordan, 1992; Walker, 1998), a person may experience reduced receptivity to connection; that is, he or she may mediate relationships primarily through strategies of disconnection (Walker & Miller, 2000).

Empathy

Movement out of isolation into growth-fostering relationship is enabled fundamentally by the development of *empathy*. Profound respect is the foundation of empathy. From that base the therapist is better able to sustain the moment-to-moment awareness that supports action in relationship. Jordan (2002) has described empathy as a complex cognitive–affective skill that involves the ability to join with another in his or her experience, while maintaining cognitive clarity about the source of the arousal. It follows that the capacity to access one's own affects contributes to this ability (p. 235). The emphasis on empathy is certainly not unique to the relational–cultural model. However, the model does incorporate a significant attitudinal shift. In many models empathy is relegated to a supporting role—a way of laying a basis for the "real" work of transference interpretation or intrapsychic conflict resolution (Jordan, 2000). Viewed in this way, empathy may devolve into a little more than a technique to induce the client's cooperation with the therapist's efforts to ply his or her trade. While this empathy-as-technique approach to the therapeutic relationship may generate benign rapport, it is unidirectional and deterministic. Undoubtedly, this approach to empathy can result in an "I-feel-your-pain" caricature of connection. Moreover, it may give rise to idealizations that are impossible to achieve in real relationships. Jordan (2002) maintains that the process of empathic joining allows access to another's subjective experience; however, perfect congruence is unattainable. The primary work of relational–cultural therapy is movement into healing connection, and Jordan (2000) suggests that empathy is itself a healing aspect of this process. In the process of empathic joining, the "real" work of therapy happens as a person moves out of isolation and comes to view him- or herself as worthy of respect and connection.

Mutual Empathy

Jordan (2002) compellingly argues that *mutual empathy* is key in moving a relationship toward deeper and more resilient connection. That is, not only must the therapist have a capacity to be moved by the client, he or she must be willing to demonstrate that response in the actual relationship. However, the therapist's ability to take in the cognitive and affective aspects of the client's experience, though essential, cannot facilitate growthful change, in and of itself. The client must know that not only can the therapist "take in" his or her experience, but also that this experience actually *matters* in the relationship with the therapist. Given the understanding that isolation is a primal source of human suffering, the therapist's failure to acknowledge the client's impact may trigger feelings of shame and relational ineptitude in the client—perhaps similar to previous experiences of being in the presence of a more powerful, nonresponsive person. Mutual empathy requires the therapist's willingness to move information (i.e., the information of his or her response to the client) out, into the relationship, rather than conceal it behind a mask of neutrality. Miller (2002) emphasizes the importance of mutual empathy in therapy because it enables clients to know that they can have an impact on the world, specifically on the people who are important in their world. Because this sense of impact may have been missing in the past, mutual empathy is viewed as a vital corrective experience in that it contributes to clients' sense of empowerment and to therapists' capacity for new learning.

Authenticity

Throughout this text, the reader will witness the therapist grappling with issues of *authenticity*. Each case poses dilemmas that require the therapist to consider key questions, such as:

1. What constitutes authentic responsiveness?
2. What are the enabling conditions and the inhibitive factors for authenticity?
3. How will authenticity facilitate movement toward healing connection at critical junctures in the relationship?

Miller and her colleagues (1999) have described authenticity as an increasing capacity for representing oneself more fully in relationship. It signals respect for the complexity of each person, acknowledges the importance of embodied difference, and invites expression of that difference in relationship (Walker, 2002). Given the premise that psychological growth is a function of action in relationship, it follows that authenticity is a critical process in relational–cultural therapy. Those aspects of self-experience that remain locked out of relationship are unavailable for growth and are susceptible to what Miller (1988) has termed "condemned isolation."

Much care is taken to distinguish authenticity from gratuitous or reactive disclosure. Authenticity is not an impulsive "tell-all" reaction. Neither is it disclosure upon demand. Indeed ill-timed or self-serving expressions of "honesty" may, in fact, result in increased shame, entrapment, and disconnection. In contrast, authenticity requires that disclosure be guided by considerations of purpose, timeliness, and capacity. The therapist must exercise judgment to discern the criteria for therapeutic disclosure: what, when, and how information might be used to promote growthful change. Moreover, it is critical to understand that disclosure is only one aspect of authenticity. First and foremost, authenticity denotes a quality of presence and availability in relationship (J. V. Jordan, personal communication, March 7, 2003). In the cases that follow, the authors demonstrate the importance of empathic attunement and relational accountability (Walker, 2002) as they work to facilitate movement toward authentic connection.

Therapist Vulnerability Reframed

Related to the process of increasing authentic responsiveness is the issue of *therapist vulnerability*. In the dominant culture, vulnerability is often seen as a danger to be minimized, if not outright avoided. Indeed, the implicit message in many traditional training settings is that therapist vulnerability is evidence of therapist ineptitude. It is small wonder, then, that the relationship between client and therapist is often constructed to fix the client as the sole repository of vulnerability. When vulnerability is viewed only as danger, there is increased likelihood of shaming in the relationship. Since the client typically holds less power in the relationship, he or she is likely to bear the brunt of the shame. The relational–cultural model reframes vulnerability to emphasize the importance of nonjudging awareness and self-empathy, qualities that allow the therapist to view his or her uncertainty as an opportunity for growth in his or her own capacity for sustaining the complexity inherent in connection. Making oneself vulnerable signals trust and respect, as does receiving and honoring the vulnerability of another (Lawrence-Lightfoot, 2000, p. 93).

As the cases illustrate, awareness of therapist vulnerability does not imply that the therapist should hijack the relationship to serve his or her own needs. Nor does it connote any lessening of therapist responsibility for expending his or her best efforts in the clients' behalf. The therapist should possess special knowledge, and he or she must exercise that knowledge in the client's behalf. However, relational–cultural practitioners also recognize that expertise is fluid (Fletcher, 1999). Such recognition releases the therapist from idealized (and shaming) images of perfection and unwavering certainty. He or she is then free to relate to the client in active and alive ways, experiencing him- or herself more as a real person-therapist than as a therapist-impersonator.

Mutuality

The relational–cultural model has always emphasized *mutuality*. Surrey (1991) asserts that mutuality is a fundamental property of healthy, growth-enhancing connections and describes it as a creative process in which the contributions of each person and openness to change allow something new to happen. Conventional usage of the word *mutuality* tends to connote reciprocity, which implies sameness. However, relational–cultural therapy makes no presumption about sameness, nor does it assign equal responsibility to the client for facilitating movement in the relationship. In fact, Surrey expressly states that the specific focus and primary purpose of the therapy relationship is the growth and healing of the client through elucidation of the client's experience (1991, p. 10). Additionally, it is essential that the relationship proceed with clarity about power relations: how power is constructed in relationship, how it is used, and for what purposes. Miller (1976) has noted that in most instances of difference, there is inequal power and that it is often normative practice for those with more power to treat those with less power destructively. In relational–cultural practice, it is the therapist's obligation to be mindful of that differential and to work assiduously to (1) prevent its potentially deleterious effects, and to (2) facilitate movement that reduces its impact on the relationship. This movement cannot occur unless the therapist is open to being influenced by the client.

Power in Relationships

Relational–cultural therapy, like all therapy practiced in the United States, takes place within a culture that is characterized by inequal distributions of power. Miller and Stiver (1991) have defined power as the capacity to produce change. This definition suggests that power is a fundamental energy of everyday living. However, in a culture that overvalorizes separation and deterministic control, this power may readily mutate into *power over* others. A *power-over culture*, as Miller (1976) defines it, is one where those with more power act in ways that maintain the power differential, undermining any movement that threatens the status quo. Moreover, the powerful behave in ways that engender conflict but simultaneously move to suppress its expression in relationship. The powerful oppose movement toward shared power while obscuring the function and intent of their actions. Traditional psychotherapies arise from this larger culture. Miller is clear that the whole therapy arrangement augments the therapist's power and can easily replicate the functions of the power-over culture from which it arises. For this reason, she posits the importance of sharing *power with* the client. As she and Stiver (1997) elucidated this point in *The Healing Connection*, the client is viewed as a supplicant—the one with problems; he or she is in a "one down" position in relation to the therapist. He or she enters the therapist's domain, where the rules of encounter, such as those about "boundaries" and "therapist neutrality," may be rigidly prescribed and held (W. B. Rosen, personal communication, June 2002). Most important, the patient may feel in more need of the relationship than the therapist. To the extent that the client experiences him- or herself as the person who "cares the most" about the relationship, he or she may feel at a great disadvantage in terms of power (Miller, 2002). It is the therapist's responsibility to be present in the relationship in ways that minimize the potentially shaming impact of such felt powerlessness. To that end, helping the client to see his or her impact on the relationship becomes an essential curative process.

In relational–cultural therapy, the therapist is responsible for ensuring that the inherent power differentials do not result in an abuse of power. Some of the practices conventionally associated with therapy can function as little more that reenactments of power-over arrangements. An example of such an arrangement is that of therapist neutrality. Rarely does one human being engage in an intense encounter with another and remain neutral throughout the process. To assume such a stance in therapy is simply disingenuous. That the values of nonresponsive neutrality and empathic possibility would be held simultaneously is one of the mystifications of modern therapy that relational–cultural practice seeks to rectify. Although the presumed benefit to the client is to allow therapeutic transference to emerge, Jordan (2000, 2002) contends that nonresponsive neutrality may, in fact, be iatrogenic, undermining movement toward relational empowerment for both client and therapist. The supposedly neutral stance masks and expands the therapist's privilege. It is as if the therapist dons a cloak of invisibility and is thereby able to hide from view the ways in which his or her own thoughts and feelings are socially inflected. Worse, according to Miller and Stiver (1997), the client may actually reexperience the ways in which he or she was left feeling powerless and isolated in the presence of a powerful, unyielding Other.

Boundary Issues

The issue of *boundaries* is central to any discussion about the construction of power in the therapy relationship. The stance that distinguishes relational–cultural practice from many traditional models is the belief that boundaries represent a place of meeting and exchange rather than a line of rigid demarcation (Jordan, 2000). The concept of boundaries tends to carry connotations of separateness and deterministic control. It is the therapist who has the power to establish the boundaries, the terms and conditions of the relationship. Although practitioners of relational–cultural therapy are wary of language that implies separateness and objectification, they are concerned with the ongoing process of establishing relational clarity. In each case presented in this book, the author must discern how the clarifying process contributes to ethical and effective practice. A central aspect of ethical practice in relational–cultural therapy is the diminution of unnecessary power differentials. The model stipulates that some power differentials are necessary (Miller, 1976). For example, teachers generally have more power than students, and parents typically have more power than children because of the presumably greater knowledge, experience, and obligation that teachers or parents have. However, the purpose of those relationships is to facilitate growth in ways that reduce or eliminate the power differential. When the therapist can act unilaterally (and in perpetuity) to establish the terms and conditions of relationship, serious questions about power arise.

Relational–cultural theorists (Jordan, 2002; Miller, 2003) have proposed a set of explicit practices to counteract the misuse of boundaries to preserve unnecessary power differentials. For example, if a client persistently seeks extrasession contact with the therapist, Jordan maintains that the therapist has an obligation to state relational limits as well as his or her own personal limitations. By doing so, he or she is taking appropriate care of the therapeutic process as well as appropriate responsibility for his or her own limitations. Moreover, the therapist avoids pathologizing the client for making a request that he or she (the therapist) is uncomfortable granting. The relational–cultural model recognizes the importance of stating limits, limitations, and agreements. Clarifying the terms of the relationship *with* the client helps to protect the relationship from destructive enactments of power. Indeed, the process of clarifying the terms may open channels of meaning, communication, and exchange. To that end, relational–cultural theory practitioners are vigilant observers of process who distinguish between agreements that promote clarity and boundaries that mystify the nature of the relationship and preserve the therapist's power over the client.

As these considerations indicate, the relational–cultural practitioner has an ethical obligation to discern what is actually being protected and at whose expense. Miller (2002) has noted that the therapist carries most of the power in the relationship and bears responsibility for its appropriate use: Specifically, the therapist should not use his or her power to secure more and lasting power over the client. In much traditional practice, the client must participate in the relationship according to terms unilaterally determined by the therapist. To counteract this norm, Miller (2003) suggests that the therapist should take explicit steps to minimize the risk of misusing the power differential. To this end, Miller has proposed that the therapist initiate a conversation with the client at the beginning of the relationship about mutual agreements: the terms and conditions that both parties need in order to make the relationship work. In the absence of these explicit agreements, boundaries, as they are traditionally constructed, will likely accrue more to the benefit of the boundary maker—the therapist—than to the relationship.

When boundaries are unilateral determinations that protect the therapist's power, the relationship loses some of its capacity for responsiveness. This boundaries-as-protection attitude casts power in win/lose terms: by implication, the relationship then becomes adversarial, with each participant struggling to maintain his or her share of a limited (and therefore more "prized") commodity. This attitude toward power often results in practices that restrict empathic possibilities and undermine movement toward mutuality.

In contrast, relational–cultural theory conceptualizes power as a shared energy of relationship, a quality that facilitates productive movement (Miller, 1976). Although when the relationship typically begins, the therapist is in a position of *power over* the client, the very function of the relational–cultural therapeutic relationship is to move toward shared *power with* the client. As the following cases illustrate, it is critical for the therapist to discern whether boundaries support clarity in relationship or defensive protection of his or her power over the client. At all times, it is important for the therapist to make legitimate use of the power the therapeutic relationship affords. To do less would be to abdicate his or her responsibility. To aid in these considerations, Surrey (1991) has these identified key questions by which therapists can evaluate a specific boundary-related practice:

- What is the potential impact of the practice on the client, the therapist, and the relationship?
- Will the behavior move the relationship toward expanded connection, either by increasing the likelihood of empathic joining or by encouraging the client to embrace a challenge?
- How does the practice affect the therapist's ability to be present to, and responsive in, relationship?

The type of discernment process these questions promote supports intentionality and accountability, thus enabling the therapist to move from a default position of *power over* to *power with* the client.

Cultural Controlling Images

One of the ways power is constructed in any culture is through the proliferation of *controlling images*. Coined by Patricia Hill Collins (1990), the term describes culturally constructed "stories" about groups and individuals that communicate how that group or individual is to be regarded by others. Collins puts it well: Controlling images are falsities that have the effect of holding people in place; that is, they protect existing objectifications and power arrangements. In psychotherapy traditions, as in the broader culture, controlling images provide much the same function as stereotypes; that is, they are used to justify particular patterns or modes of relationship (Allport, 1954). More than a set of abstract beliefs, these images have social as well as emotional significance. As such, they are never politically neutral; they most often serve the interests of those who are socially empowered by denigrating people who are culturally marginalized. For example, Collins identified controlling images associated with American black females, such as "Welfare Queen" and "Mammy." The images function as a kind cognitive–affective code for apprehending relational possibility. As such, they may result in objectifications that foreclose empathic awareness and movement toward mutuality. Reflective of the dominant society in which it is embedded, the culture of therapy also proliferates controlling images that may constrain movement in relationship. For example, the image of the therapist as Unfailingly Wise or Perpetually Empathic imposes a set of shaming idealizations that may constrict the therapist's openness to new learning in relationship. Similarly, there exist many disempowering controlling images associated with clients. Many of the Axis II diagnostic labels so readily applied to clients (e.g., borderline) serve as a ready-made explanations for disturbances in relationship. When used in this manner, these explanations preclude a quality of presence and responsiveness in relationship that would allow the therapist and client to do the hard and risky work of making change.

Personal Relational Images

In many of the cases that follow, the authors are consciously exploring the link between controlling images and *relational images*. Miller and Stiver (1995, 1997) define relational images as "key inner concepts used to order experience." These concepts are derived from past experiences with others and determine, to a large extent, our beliefs about why relationships are as they are. The relational images form a framework through which meaning is created, expectation is formed, and relational worthiness is established. Miller and Stiver (1997) suggest that the explanations we create about relationships form the basis of our story about how we must function in the world: who we are, how we are regarded by others, who others are, as well as what we can expect from, and deserve to receive in, a relationship. Simply put, relational images provide the template for what informs us of what we must be or do in order to find connection (Miller & Stiver, 1997).

Much of the work of therapy involves the transformation of relational images. Similar to the concept of cognitive schema associated with Beckian and other cognitive models, relational images may trigger repetitive reenactments and inhibit psychological growth. However, in relational–cultural practice, the clinician works to uncover the link between the "inner working model" of the individual and the outer workings of the broader culture. When the client and clinician enter the therapeutic relationship, they bring with them not only their personal developmental histories but also the cultural history of the groups with which they are socially identified. As the cases in this volume demonstrate, relational images that are enacted in particular relationships are often aligned with, or are derivative of, the controlling images associated with their cultural histories. Because of the distorted power arrangements inherent in controlling images, this alignment results in severely attenuated receptivity to mutual engagement in relationship. When relational images are aligned with the controlling images of the dominant culture, both client and therapist are prone to defensive enactments. These enactments are attempts to "survive" the relationship through strategies of disconnection, rather than engage it through authentic connection. In fact, much of what is termed *transference* in traditional models refers to these enactments. As Stiver (1991b) explains, transference is very much a relational phenomenon in which the connections and disconnections of past relationships are enacted—often symbolically and without awareness. A therapeutic relationship characterized by empathic possibility, authentic responsiveness, and felt mutuality provides the safety for the images to emerge—and emerge, they must, for otherwise they remain underground, preserving the distortions that inhibit empowering movement and possibility. In the process of emergence, both client and therapist gain a greater understanding of the chronic disconnections that lead to suffering and isolation.

Opening oneself to the possibility for transformation is a profound act of courage. It is the work of relational–cultural therapy. In that sense, the relational–cultural theory model challenges deep biases in the dominant culture, as well as in the culture of traditional therapy (J. V. Jordan, personal communication, February 25, 2003). Both client and therapist are carriers and preservers of images—images that are often too small to contain the complexity of their experience in relationship. As is revealed in the cases that follow, the therapy relationship challenges both client and therapist to relinquish the images that provide an illusory certainty and safety in relationship. Irene Stiver, a beloved founding scholar who died in September 2000, often spoke of the faith required to embrace the risks of complexity in order to experience the fulfillment of growthful change. Relational–cultural therapy encourages action in relationship: empathic attunement to emergent experience and openness to movement through mutual influence. Audre Lorde, feminist activist and poet, described this process in a letter to her therapist when she wrote: "some part of my journey is yours too" (1984). The authors of these case narratives reveal the complexity of those journeys. Guided by the principles of relational–cultural theory, they tell stories that offer hope for an expanded vision of human possibility: stories that illuminate the journey toward the emergence of something new.

REFERENCES

Allport, G. (1954). *The nature of prejudice*. Cambridge, MA: Addison-Wesley.

Broverman, I., Broverman, D., Clarkson, F., Rosenkrantz, P., & Vogel, S. (1970). Sex role stereotypes and clinical judgments of mental health. *Journal of Consulting and Counseling Psychology, 43,* 1–7.

Collins, P. H. (1990). *Black feminist thought: Knowledge, consciousness, and the politics of empowerment*. Boston: Unwin Hyman.

Fletcher, J. K. (1999). *Disappearing acts: Gender, power, and relational practice at work*. Cambridge, MA: MIT Press.

Freud, S. (1955). Beyond the pleasure principle. In J. S. Strachey (Ed. & Trans.), *The standard edition of the complete psychological works of Sigmund Freud* (Vol. 18, pp. 3–64). London: Hogarth Press. (Original work published 1920)

Gilligan, C. (1982). *In a different voice*. Boston: Harvard University Press.

hooks, b. (1984). *Feminist theory: From margin to center*. Boston: South End Press.

Jordan, J. V. (2000). The role of mutual empathy in relational–cultural therapy. *Journal of Clinical Psychology/In Session: Psychotherapy in Practice, 56*(80), 1005–1016.

Jordan, J. V. (2001). A relational–cultural model: Healing through mutual empathy. *Bulletin of the Menninger Clinic, 65*(1), 92–103

Jordan, J. V. (2002) A relational–cultural perspective in therapy. In F. Kaslow *Comprehensive handbook of psychotherapy* (Vol. 3, pp. 233–254). New York: Wiley.

Jordan, J. V., Surrey, J. C., & Kaplan, A. G. (1991). Women and empathy: Implications for psychological development and psychotherapy. In J. V. Jordan, A. G. Kaplan, J. B. Miller, I. P. Stiver, & J. L. Surrey (Eds.), *Women's growth in connection: Writings from the Stone Center* (pp. 27–50). New York: Guilford Press.

Jordan, J. V., & Hartling, L. M. (2002). New developments in relational–cultural theory. In M. Ballou & L. S. Brown (Eds.), *Rethinking mental health and disorder: Feminist perspectives* (pp. 48–70). New York: Guilford Press.

Jordan, J. V., Kaplan, A., Miller, J. B., Stiver, I. P., & Surrey J. L. (1991). *Women's growth in connection: Writings from the Stone Center*. New York: Guilford Press.

Kaplan, A. (1991). How can a group of white, heterosexual, privileged women claim to speak of "women's" experience? In J. B. Miller, J. V. Jordan, A. G. Kaplan, I. P. Stiver, & J. L. Surrey (Eds.), Some misconceptions and reconceptions of a relational approach. *Work in Progress, No. 49* (pp. 5–7). Wellesley, MA: Stone Center Working Paper Series.

Lawrence-Lightfoot, S. (2000). *Respect: An exploration*. New York: Perseus.

Lorde, A. (1984). *Sister outsider: Speeches and essays*. Freedom, CA: Crossing Press.

Miller, J. B. (1976). *Toward a new psychology of women*. Boston: Beacon Press.

Miller, J. B. (1984). The development of women's sense of self. *Work in Progress, No. 12.*. Wellesley, MA: Stone Center Working Paper Series.

Miller, J. B. (1988). Connections, disconnections, and violations. *Work in Progress, No. 33*. Wellesley, MA: Stone Center Working Paper Series.

Miller, J. B. (2002). How change happens: Controlling images, mutuality, and power. *Works in Progress, No. 96*. Wellesley, MA: Stone Center Working Paper Series.

Miller, J. B. (2003). Telling the truth about power. *Work in Progress, No. 100*. Wellesley, MA: Stone Center Working Paper Series.

Miller, J. B., Jordan, J. V., Stiver, I. P., Walker, M., Surrey, J. L., & Eldridge, N. S. (1999). Therapist's authenticity. *Work in Progress, No. 82*. Wellesley, MA: Stone Center Working Paper Series.

Miller, J. B., & Stiver, I. P. (1991). A relational reframing of therapy. *Work in Progress, No. 52*. Wellesley, MA: Stone Center Working Paper Series.

Miller, J. B., & Stiver, I. (1995). Relational images and their meanings in psychotherapy. *Work in Progress, No. 74*. Wellesley, MA: Stone Center Working Paper Series.

Miller, J. B., & Stiver, I. P. (1997). *The healing connection*. Boston: Beacon Press.

Spencer, R. (2000). A comparison of relational psychologies. *Project Report, No. 5*. Wellesley, MA: Stone Center Series.

Stiver, I. P. (1990). Dysfunctional families and wounded relationship: Part 1. *Work in Progress, No. 41*. Wellesley, MA: Stone Center Working Paper Series.

Stiver, I. P. (1991a). The meaning of care: Reframing treatment models. In J. V. Jordan, A. G. Kaplan, J. B. Miller, I. P. Stiver, & J. L. Surrey (Eds.), *Women's growth in connection: Writings from the Stone Center* (pp. 250–267). New York: Guilford Press.

Stiver, I. P. (1991b). What is the role of transference and the unconscious in the relational model? In J. B. Miller, J. V. Jordan, A. G. Kaplan, I. P. Stiver, & J. L. Surrey (Eds.), Some misconceptions and reconceptions of a relational approach. *Work in Progress, No. 49* (pp. 8–10). Wellesley, MA: Stone Center Working Paper Series.

Stiver, I. P. (1992). A relational approach to therapeutic impasse. *Work in Progress, No. 58*. Wellesley, MA: Stone Center Working Paper Series.

Surrey, J. L. (1991). "What do you mean by mutuality in therapy?" In J.B. Miller, J.V. Jordan, A. G. Kaplan, I.P. Stiver, & J.L. Surrey (Eds.) *Some misconceptions and reconceptions of a relational approach*. Work in Progress, No. 49, Wellesley, MA: Stone Center Working Paper Series

Walker, M. (1998). Race, self, and society: Relational challenges in a culture of disconnection. *Work in Progress, No. 85.* Wellesley, MA: Stone Center Working Paper Series.

Walker, M. (2002). How therapy helps when the culture hurts. *Work in Progress, No. 95.* Wellesley, MA: Stone Center Working Paper Series.

Walker, M., & Miller, J. B. (2001). Racial images and relational possibilities. *Talking Paper, No. 2.* Wellesley, MA: Stone Center Talking Paper Series.

2

Relational Learning in Psychotherapy Consultation and Supervision

JUDITH V. JORDAN

 T here are some who would argue that psychotherapy cannot be taught, that therapists are born, not made. Others suggest that therapy is an entirely skill- and theory-based practice that can be taught systematically. As with so many of our binary constructions, neither speaks to the wholeness and complexity of becoming a therapist. Most approaches to teaching psychotherapy, however divergent the core concepts, involve a relationship between a student and a supervisor, a form of relational learning.

RELATIONAL–CULTURAL THERAPY: WORKING WITH CONNECTION AND DISCONNECTION

The relational–cultural model suggests that isolation is the primary source of suffering for people, and it proposes that we grow and heal in connection rather than by becoming more autonomous or separate. Jean Baker Miller and Irene Stiver have outlined the course of this healing in *The Healing Connection* (1997). Other basic tenets of the work were put forth in Jordan and colleagues' *Women's Growth in Connection* (1991),

Women's Growth in Diversity (1997), and in the approximately 100 *Works in Progress* that have been published at the Stone Center since 1981. As noted in Chapter 1, the core processes that are assumed to create change or growth in people are mutual empathy, relational authenticity, and mutual empowerment. Jean Baker Miller has written about the five good things (zest, clarity, increased sense of worth, creativity/productivity, and desire for more connection) that occur in all growth-fostering relationships.

Acute disconnections occur ubiquitously in relationships when one person misunderstands, injures, or violates another person. These injuries need not be intentional, nor need they be permanently damaging. In fact, when the injured person can represent his or her needs and feelings to the other person and feels responded to—as if his or her feelings matter to the other person—he or she is empowered, feels relationally competent, and the relationship is strengthened. In order for relational resilience to develop, the more powerful person must indicate that he or she cares about the feelings and experience of the less powerful person and has an interest in reworking the disconnection. The reworking of disconnections actually strengthens people's connections and affirms their ability to create those connections—to have an effect on others.

Chronic disconnections occur when, in an important ongoing relationship (particularly when it is characterized by inequal power distribution), the less powerful person is not responded to or is unable to represent his or her needs and feelings. The more powerful person may respond with avoidance, denial, shaming, or attack. In such interactions the less powerful person is silenced, feels relationally incompetent (he or she cannot move or affect the other person or the relationship), and feels unable to bring him- or herself authentically into the relationship. The less powerful person moves into what Jean Baker Miller calls "condemned isolation" (Miller & Stiver, 1997); the relationship begins to lose its vitality, mutuality, and depth. This downward spiral leaves the less powerful person feeling vulnerable, ineffective, incompetent, isolated, and possibly endangered. If these interactions are repeated over time with an important and powerful other person (e.g., a parent, older sibling, partner), they will generalize (as relational images) in such a way that all relationships will be experienced as potentially limiting rather than growth fostering.

The work of therapy, largely through mutual empathy, is to help bring the client back into a place of connection where healthy psychological growth can occur once again. Relational images shift, hope develops, and a belief in the positive power of connection emerges; the client feels less isolated. Not only does empathy create better understanding of a person, it also provides an experiential sense of being "joined with," of moving out of isolation. In order for empathy to create change, however, it must be mutual. When mutual empathy is present, the client sees, knows, and feels that the therapist is responsive to, and moved by, his or her experience. Mutual empathy provides a sense of relational effectiveness and joining, and it facilitates the development of new relational images in which vulnerability and authenticity become safer prospects, and the person is able to begin to represent more and more of his or her experience in this healing relationship. Eventually all relational images begin to shift, and empathic possibility begins to emerge in other relationships. The use of mutual empathy in therapy challenges many of the more traditional dynamic approaches that emphasize therapist objectivity, neutrality, or nongratification in the therapeutic relationship.

In order for therapists to participate in mutually empathic, healing relationships, they must learn to work with their own responsiveness, their own empathic attunement, as well as their own movement toward disconnection. A therapist's growth is best facilitated in supervision that is itself characterized by mutual empathy and nonjudgmental and nonshaming interactions. In this context supervision can provide similar experiences of change and growth.

MUTUAL EMPATHY IN SUPERVISION AND THERAPY

Many people express uneasiness about how mutual empathy works and how it can be developed in therapists. As noted in Chapter 1, mutual empathy is not about reciprocal empathy (i.e., you empathize with me, and then I'll empathize with you, reciprocally); it is not about the therapist's self-disclosure of personal facts; it is not a denial of the therapist's professional role, which involves ethical and legal standards; it is not a denial of the power differential between therapist and client. It is about real engagement and real responsiveness, not knee-jerk reactivity or total spontaneity. The therapist's responses are guided by a dedication to doing what promotes the healing and well-being of the client. This model of authenticity and engagement involves a delicate, thoughtful process of being real while also being guided by clinical judgment. It is, as Irene Stiver pointed out, finding the "one true thing" (the piece of what is true that can be shared) that can be said to facilitate movement in the relationship and growth in the client. The therapist is guided by principles of the relational–cultural model, anticipatory empathy, and the ethical principles of his or her professional group. Based on an understanding of, and deep respect for, the client and his or her relational resources, together with an appreciation of how mutuality develops, the therapist finds ways to engage the client that allow the client to see how he or she affects the therapist, that his or her feelings matter, and that he or she does not have to suffer alone. Active understanding of the client's patterns of disconnection and strategies for survival, together with empathy for the suffering experienced due to shame, self-blame, and isolation, serve to help the client feel heard and seen.

WORKING WITH SHAME AND VULNERABILITY

For mutual empathy to develop in therapists, it is essential that supervision be conducted in an atmosphere that is safe, respectful, and based on a model of mutual learning. Too often the supervisor is seen as all knowing (and sometimes acts that way). It is important that the supervisor respect the supervisee's vulnerability in this situation. According this respect means that the supervisor must also work with his or her own vulnerability. Supervisors must be extremely sensitive to possible issues of shame in supervisees, just as therapists must be aware of this potential with clients. Too often, in a field characterized by much opinion that passes for scientific truth, new therapists are ashamed of their uncertainty, the extent to which they do not feel confident about their interventions, and their own human limitations. Although all supervisors have a responsibility to provide thoughtful and corrective feedback, particularly when they feel that a student may be proceeding in an unwise or hurtful direction with a client, it is also incumbent on supervisors to find respectful and empathic ways to offer their critiques. Stories abound of the harsh, shaming responses from supervisors to supervisees. Often supervisees are shamed for having "poor boundaries" if they practice in a more responsive, relational way. Supervisors are obliged to find ways to encourage growth-promoting psychotherapy practice that does not humiliate or shame the students. The lack of immediate validation and the degree of complexity and uncertainty in the healing process make it especially important that we proceed with utmost respect and humility as supervisors, and that the supervisory process itself is collaborative and characterized by "fluid expertise"(Fletcher, 1999).

Shaming can occur unwittingly when supervisors are not attuned to power dynamics in the supervisory relationship or in the larger culture. Some supervisors proceed with little awareness of social forces of stratification and marginalization, as if individuals exist in a vacuum. Supervisees, partly because they are in positions of less power, sometimes are not free to represent their own perspectives (e.g., as a woman, as a person of color, as a lesbian or gay therapist). Supervision should be characterized by fluid expertise. Many supervisors trained in largely intrapsychic models may have difficulty taking into account the cultural, sociopolitical forces that disempower and isolate both clients and supervisees.

Since the relational–cultural model does not depend on a systematic set of techniques, it poses particular problems when we try to teach/ supervise. I believe that the therapy relationship is unique, and that there is much to learn in the practice of therapy. In fact, I believe that the learning is lifelong, and that all of us should be in some form of supervision or consultation for our entire careers. I also think we learn about growth-fostering relationships not only in therapy but in all our relationships (and hopefully practice the principles there too). With new therapists, we may have to err a bit on the side of pointing out the differences between the therapeutic relationship and ordinary social relationships. Initial supervisory tasks include the provision of thoughtfulness and respect, "holding" the goal of helping the client change, and guiding the supervisee to step into a professional helping role that is imbued with authentic responsiveness. Reading and talking about principles and theory and looking at clinical dilemmas are an important part of developing competence and confidence. It is important that supervisors share their learning experiences, their hard times as well as their successes. If the supervisee has been trained in a more traditional mode, some rethinking and unlearning must occur, particularly if that mode includes the old "blank screen" approach and those that suggest the therapist's emotional responsiveness is only a burden for the client.

It is essential that we, as clinicians, maintain the capacity to be present, to connect, to become aware of the forces of disconnection and vulnerability, and to learn *with* our clients. Clearly our own places of disconnection become problematic if we do not work with them. We must (1) be aware of the disconnections, (2) try to figure out their source (in ourselves, the other, or in the dynamics of this particular relationship), (3) move into an inner space of interest and curiosity (rather than defensiveness and withdrawal) around the disconnection, and (4) then share our understandings in a nonshaming way when the time is right. This reflective process suggests the capacity to stay in our vulnerability and to move back into connection, rather than adopting a "one up" or power over position. Working with a kind of relational resilience, we are able to "move," to respond, rather than become caught in images of what we "should be." These "ideal self" images are prevalent in life, in general (e.g., "I should be mature, popular, smart, cool," etc.) and virtually rampant in therapists and supervisors (e.g., "I should have my own problems all worked out," "I should be connecting and relational at all times," "I should be completely generous and kind in thought, word, and deed," etc.). Supervision can reinforce all these images, leading to extensive silencing of the supervisee, or it can provide a place of safety where people can explore and understand how these images function in their therapy work. When supervision reinforces unrealistic images of how a therapist or supervisor must function, the supervisee often develops a sense of isolation, of being alone with the difficult task of "learning" psychotherapy. Often this atmosphere occurs in a larger teaching context that is shaming, built on "separate self" and "certainty" models of functioning and learning. Although supervision that appears to offer absolute truths and "answers" has an appeal, particularly for beginning students, it often leads to feelings of fraudulence (in both the supervisor and supervisee), to shame for less than "perfect" functioning, and to isolation (a worry that if one were really known or one's work were truly seen, one would be judged negatively and rejected). The learning of therapy and supervision depends on an attitude of openness and flexibility, an awareness of one's own patterns of disconnection, and a readiness to stand in uncertainty. I would like to turn now, not to a supervised case, but to a *supervision experience* in which I have been learning and growing, as "consultant."

SUPERVISION GROUP

Irene Stiver and I ran a supervision/consultation group using the relational–cultural model from 1991 until the time of her death in 2000. Since her death, I have continued as consultant to the group. This is a group for experienced therapists who have been trained in more traditional psychodynamic models but who have also read widely in the relational–cultural literature. Group members include psychologists, social workers, and psychiatric nurses; most are in private practice, several have medical school appointments and work part time in hospital programs, and one recently became active in politics as an elected official.

Irene and I initially decided to conduct this group when she was leaving her position at a Harvard teaching hospital, where we had worked together (in addition to working on the development of Stone Center theory). We both loved working together (she was first my mentor, and then my valued colleague, and it seems like she was always a best friend). The group initially met a real need for us: It provided a regular way to work together, to deepen our thinking—and to give us an excuse for lunch every other week. We felt dedicated to helping other practitioners gain "hands-on" experience with relational–cultural therapy, and we expected to learn with and from them. The group of six women met weekly, and we rotated case presentations so that in each 1½ hour session, two people presented cases (45 minutes each). Each week Irene and I traded the function of time keeper and detail person (e.g., announcements, arranging future meetings, etc.), but we both actively responded to the material presented, as did all the members of the group. We called it a consultation group rather than a supervision group (consultation felt a bit more collaborative, less authoritarian, and also reflected our practice). Once a month (or slightly less, depending on the press of clinical material) we set aside a meeting for a topic/discussion. Irene and I would typically lead these discussions, but all members participated actively. Topics included areas such as the nature of mutual empathy, the differences between relational–cultural practice and other models, how to think about transference, integrating other modalities with relational–cultural work, and the times when we just do not feel connected with our clients. Although we did not include a formal check-in procedure, the first 5–10 minutes of each meeting was often spent catching up with each other's lives: grandchildren, serious illness, deaths in our families, happy events, political or social concerns, job changes, trips, good conferences we had attended. These were not long discussions, but they had the effect of acknowledging our life issues and showing care.

When we shifted into the consultations, the designated presenter would begin by framing a concern, interest, or question. Often the cases presented contained some area of unclarity or difficulty for the therapist (members were there to get help), but sometimes they were interesting or puzzling but not troubling. Then there were always the crises about which people urgently needed to talk. These were not formal presentations but rather summaries and descriptions of particular instances in which the therapist needed some help. We listened to one another during the presentation, asking questions but mostly listening at first. As the presentation ended, we responded with feelings, thoughts, more questions, sharing similar experiences from our own practices, and noting what had "worked" for us. Occasionally we elaborated on the bigger picture: how this element of this case illustrated the difficulty of honoring the paradox of connection or disconnection, or how hard it could be at times to stay connected. One of us might share what we had originally learned to do in a similar dilemma and how we handled it differently now. These "differentiating" moments were often filled with zest, and they validated others' as well as our own growth experiences. Sometimes we suggested other resources (e.g., "Have you thought of recommending Alanon or AA?" or "I know a great group for people recovering from the loss of a spouse"). But sometimes we were just "with" each other in the difficult places. At times we had to help each other pay attention to how "stressed out" we were about a particular client issue, and we had to check in about each other's well-being in the face of a particular clinical stressor. There was clearly an interest in assisting one another through the tough times and of helping one another develop a kind of relational resilience—the ability to turn to connection in the times of stress. We all served that function for one another. Although it was never a "process group," and it was always far more than a "support group," this consultation group was, and continues to be, a source of learning, support, and inspiration.

Irene and I often discussed writing about this experience; we never got to do it. But she is with me now as I try to grasp the special quality of this group. It is a compassionate group. This does not mean that we are all always very compassionate people, but there is a pervading ethic of compassion. Indeed, it is a group characterized by shared vulnerability and compassion. People give gentle feedback based on their own experiences. People present their difficulties, their "mistakes," their questions, and their sense of inadequacy. In the midst of some of the muddles, there is a deep respect for the intentions of the presenting therapist and a humble awareness of the limitations of our "knowledge" without feeling we "know nothing." And there is an appreciation of the collaborative wisdom that exists in the group, often with different individuals offering special pieces of the movement toward growth. We have created a spirit of supported vulnerability. People also present some of those wonderful moments in therapy when change happens and both client and therapist grow and expand. People sometimes disagree or are concerned about the path someone is taking, but the feedback, if critical, is offered tentatively, gently (e.g., "Have you thought about . . . " "When I've had to deal with that, I've tried . . . "). Sometimes we are all stumped by a particular challenge, and we sit with that not-knowing moment, naming the places of uncertainty. Sometimes we feel awe (and perhaps envy) at the way someone else has handled a problem. The learning is clearly and fully mutual; each of the participants has a great deal to teach the rest of us. There are times when Irene and I both felt we should have been more "expert," and we would have to remind each other of our belief in "fluid expertise" and mutual learning!

The loss of Irene had an enormous impact on the group. I felt bereft without her, and the other members profoundly missed her. But she is often with us, invoked by countless references such as, "I'll always remember when Irene said . . . " or "What do you think Irene would say?" We continue to learn about—and benefit from—the power of connection with each other, with Irene, and with other practitioners who work with the relational model. This group has empowered us, as clinicians, to listen to our own wisdom (we "listen each other into voice"), to better use the relational model in our work with clients. It helps us respond with resilience when the doubts and difficulties of therapeutic work sometimes sap our resources. Often simply coming into the group and naming a particularly hard place (e.g., "I feel so stuck") or allowing fears (e.g., "I really don't know if this is helping my client") starts the process of movement. We begin to come out of the isolation and the stuckness. The response of the leader and other group members, the empathic listening, gentle questioning, and sharing of similar dilemmas often allow each of us to reconnect with our own understanding and ultimately with our clients. This process also often facilitates a release from the hold of shaming images: "What's wrong with me if I don't know what's going on here, if I have doubt, if I get angry or secretly wish this client would quit?"; or "What's wrong if I feel I care 'too much'?" Sometimes the group has to struggle with the dilemma of giving feedback that may be difficult to hear, for instance, if one or two of the group feels that another member is extending herself too much or losing touch with her client in some way. Finding the way to register difference or concern can be a challenge. But in this group, all the members are committed to finding ways to gently share these kinds of concerns with others. On some occasions, a call to one of the leaders has helped the leader support a particular intervention or helped the member think through her own discomfort.

The group still exists. This year we have decided to try to spend a little more time on conceptual issues. We have agreed to try to pay particular attention to what contributes to change in the work we do. Although we still function as a consultation group, we are also consciously working at deepening the theoretical understandings of the relational–cultural model, both as a way to develop the theory and as a way of empowering the participants to become active creators of the work. At its best the group epitomizes the five good things of growth-fostering relationships: zest, clarity, productivity, sense of worth, and desire for more connection. At times we simply hold the intention and faith that our connection will work to create resilience and movement for both therapists and clients. We are still learning together.

REFERENCES

Fletcher, J. (1999). *Disappearing acts: Gender, power, and relational practice at work.* Cambridge, MA: MIT Press.

Jordan, J. V. (Ed.). (1997). *Women's growth in diversity: Writings from the Stone Center.* New York: Guilford Press.

Jordan, J. V., Kaplan, A. G., Miller, J. B., Stiver, I. P., & Surrey, J. L. (1991). *Women's growth in connection: More writings from the Stone Center.* New York: Guilford Press.

Miller, J. B., & Stiver, I. P. (1997). *The healing connection.* Boston: Beacon Press.

Part II

Connection, Disconnection, and Resilience in the Therapy Dyad

> Do you remember when we were growing up, and a lot of
> our families didn't have cars? You would go to visit your
> friends and when it was time to leave, they would offer to
> walk you a piece of the way.

Among black Southerners of a certain age, there is a shared memory of a custom called "walking a piece of the way." I (MW) was reminded of this custom by a client whose cultural history was very similar to my own. Her comment evoked a memory of a ritual that typically went like this. My mother and I would walk over to our cousin Corine's house for a visit. When we would leave to return home, Corine would walk with us up to some undetermined point, maybe a quarter, maybe a third, of the way back. This point was often not a place for leave taking, but for continuing the conversation. Sometimes slowly, Corine would start to wend her way back home, with my mother and me walking *her* a piece of the way back. It was not unusual for Corine to also turn at some point and walk us another piece of the way, before we each finally took our leave and headed back to those places we called home.

I have come to think of this ritual as a healing metaphor—one that represents the flow of movement in relationships where authenticity and mutual empathy are guiding precepts. It is a ritual that developed under conditions of shared material vulnerability. However, out of that vulnerability emerged deep recognition of the joy and vitality of desire that come from shared connection. To walk a piece of the way was to expose one's need and desire for relationship. In the flow of mutual influence, clarity was enhanced: Each person knew more about the other and about the relationship, and no one got lost. To walk a piece of the way with a client is to make a commitment to a level of lived complexity that many of the more tradition models of psychotherapy practice would either prohibit or ignore. For example, much of the early training of psychotherapists emphasizes the importance of a tightly bound therapeutic frame. Sometimes the accompanying admonitions very direct. One I recall is "Never leak power to the client." Read: Maintain power *over* your client lest he or she *over*power you. In most instances, therapist trainees receive not-too-subtle warnings about the undesirable consequences that ensue when the therapist allows the client to have a visible impact on his or her life. Whether direct or subtle, the advice usually translates into specific behavioral protocols, most of which function to secure most of the power in the hands of the therapist. None of this advice is ill-intentioned. Rather, it serves to create a bounded context wherein clients can engage the deep emotional wounds of their lives, undistracted by the person-hood of the therapist. However, such an emphasis on impermeable boundedness, hyperindividuation, and autonomy more likely fosters the idealization of separation and disconnection—the very forces that contribute to much of the suffering in life.

In contrast, the relational–cultural model proposes that the deepest sense of self is tied to relational movement. As Miller (1976) explains, a felt sense of self is inseparable from dynamic interaction—a precept that places relationally emergent knowing as the basis for human growth. Moreover, because the therapy relationship exists in a cultural context where power is stratified and sinuously layered along multiple dimensions, the therapist and client must pay close attention to the enactments of power between them. To attend to the cultural context of the therapy relationship is to recognize that therapy itself is a political act—one that has the potential either to reproduce the wounding disconnections of a *power-over* culture or to restore and enhance the capacity of each participant to co-create sustainable connections in the living world. Simply put, when two people come face to face in a therapy dyad, they bring not just their individual histories but the transgenerational complexities of the culture in which their lives are formed.

In the chapters that follow, the authors tell stories of complexity and resilience, pain and hope. In her narrative about a cross-racial therapy relationship with a young white college student, Walker describes her encounter with controlling, disconnecting racial images. She shows how such images can stifle creativity and inhibit healing and growth in the relationship. She also illustrates how a more relational–cultural practice might have optimized what otherwise would have been a merely satisfactory therapeutic outcome. In this first story of healing, Walker illuminates the observation often attributed to Irene Stiver: that in the therapy, movement toward image is movement out of relationship.

If therapeutic outcome is related to the therapist's capacity to embrace vulnerability and complexity, Rosen's "Making Great Memories" elucidates the possibilities that can emerge when the therapist is able to move through her own shame to encounter the client at a growing edge they both share. In this narrative, the reader is invited to ponder the ethical considerations that arise when the therapist is moved to forego some of the usual norms and strictures that mark traditional psychotherapeutic practice. Rosen guides the reader through her doubts and feeling-thoughts, and in so doing, demystifies the practices that unnecessarily reinforce the inherent inequalities of the therapy relationship.

Lawler's narrative of "Caring, but Fallible: A Story of Repairing Disconnections" illustrates the usefulness of relational–cultural practices when working with clients who exhibit complex and severe psychiatric symptomatology. In a story that is both poetic in its rendering and practical in its counsel, Lawler illustrates how the therapist must hold hope for connectedness—particularly when working with a client whose strategies of disconnection feel pointedly punitive. Lawler's narrative also demonstrates the importance of proactively developing a relational context for the therapy—a network of supportive and exacting advisors to help bear the remonstrations and self-doubt that otherwise could lead to immobilizing alienation and despair.

The fourth story in this section guides the reader through the reality of pain as it is lived by both the therapist and the client. Comstock's deep sharing in "Reflections on Life, Loss, and Resilience" allows the reader to enter the hope and possibility that lie on the other side of shame and despair. The client in this narrative is living a pain that throbs throughout her being and drives her into shame-filled isolation. She lives a pain that is well known to her therapist. With a spirit of hopefulness and belief in the power of connection, Comstock guides her client through the loss toward renewed engagement with life and loving.

The case narratives presented in this section are not simple, happy stories. They are stories of great hope. In each instance, the author illuminates her conviction that growthful movement starts with recognition of the shared incompleteness and imperfection that is the human condition. In a fashion somewhat analogous to Paulo Freire's "problem-solving education," the therapist and client work to reconcile dichotomized power arrangements that create disconnection. In other words, they recognize that the illusion of separateness is perpetuated by the vertical power arrangements that cast the client as the sole carrier of woundedness, shame, and vulnerability. As these narratives illustrate, relational–

cultural therapy affirms the process of ongoing becoming, where therapist and client alike are aware of their own vulnerability and fluidity. In the process of becoming, these therapists do not abdicate their responsibility to their clients, nor do they shirk their accountability to their professional communities. These therapists recognize that failure to exercise their expertise, however fluid, to benefit the therapy relationship is an abuse of power in itself. They recognize, too, that healing possibilities emerge through acts of co-creation, where processes of mutual empowerment continually unfold. In these therapy dyads, the client and the therapist move toward expanded relational capacity. At heart, these stories reveal works of courage by two people who are learning to walk together . . . just a piece of the way.

REFERENCE

Miller, J. B. (1976). *Toward a new psychology of women*. Boston: Beacon Press.

3

Walking a Piece of the Way

Race, Power, and
Therapeutic Movement

MAUREEN WALKER

*B*ecoming a therapist was, for me, the culmination of many life transitions. By the time I began my graduate training, I had long known that my life work would involve healing and helping others. What I did not know was how profoundly the process of becoming a therapist would require me to accept my own immediate and ongoing need for healing. As a graduate trainee, I had adopted one of the more limiting notions about therapists: that the therapist is someone who has achieved psychological stolidity—a state of near-nirvana that enables him or her to resist the emotional strains and stresses that impinge on the lives of others. I had whole-heartedly accepted the principle that the therapist should use him- or herself as an "instrument" in the service of healing others. What was problematic about this notion was the level of objectification suggested by the language of instrumentality. Specifically, I had translated "self as instrument" to mean that I should demonstrate unwavering capacity to feel for, and feel with, others. The instrument itself—the therapist—should be the perfect object: one who can be at once unwaveringly available and empathic, unfailingly wise and invulnerable. Such objectification is antithetical to relational–cultural practice, for good reason: It shrinks the therapist, making him or her less empathic with his or her own experience—and thereby less able to be present authentically in relationship, as the case I discuss in this chapter shows.

Moreover, the posture of pure instrumentality tends to disregard the fact that the therapy relationship is culturally situated. As such, it is subject to many of the same dynamics and distortions that compromise other relationships in the larger culture. It is important to be cognizant of the link, however tenuous, between the caricatured images from the popular culture and the idealized images from the culture of mainstream therapy. The popular caricature of the emotionally unflappable therapist bears a striking resemblance to the idealized image from mainstream therapy cultures. Namely, the therapist is securely bounded and self-contained, undaunted and unaffected by the distortions and uncertainties that mark intimate relationship.

In contrast, relational–cultural practice posits the centrality of mutual influence in any healing relationship. Furthermore, the model emphasizes the impact of relational embeddedness: each specific relationship, including the therapy relationship, is subject to the influence of other relationships that form its cultural context. Without conscious attention to the cultural context in which the relationship is embedded, the therapist may unwittingly replicate the cultural practices and distortions that breed disconnection. It follows that relational–cultural therapy necessarily concerns itself with questions of power: power that inheres in the structural arrangements of the therapy relationship, and power as manifest in the relational arrangements of the dominant culture. Within the context of a culture that wounds both the therapist and the client, the therapist must address the complexities inherent in the relationship, not as a perfect object-instrument, but as a co-traveler toward healing. In order for the process of mutual influence to unfold, the therapist must "show up" in relationship as an authentic presence and open him- or herself to the possibility of healing and change. As the following case narrative illustrates, to do less is to foreclose on opportunities for mutual empowerment.

This case was conducted when I was a trainee, under supervision, within a more traditional psychodynamic framework. But it is instructive to compare my handling of it at the time with my current relational–cultural therapy perspective. Walking a piece of the way seems an apt metaphor for describing the sense of presence, complexity, and mutuality that can enable therapeutic movement and enhanced relational growth.

CASE NARRATIVE

At the time of our meeting, Kira was a 20-year-old white college senior at a university where I was doing graduate training. Kira explained to me that she was seeking treatment because of occasional bouts of unhappiness, which usually involved tearful fights with her boyfriend, a man 6 years her senior. When she was 18 years old, she had decided to move in with him as a way of "managing her expenses while living in the city." As she put it, she was prone to fits of jealous rage and lived in constant fear of abandonment. Now, 2 years later, she was worried that her "moodiness" was unjustified and would eventually drive him away from her. Over the early weeks of our sessions, the content of our work shifted toward conversations about Kira's upbringing in an upper-middle-class suburban neighborhood. Her favorite description of her now-divorced parents was as a "couple of leftover hippies." Her childhood home, as she remembered it, was the site of frequent "wild parties." As the therapy progressed, it became clear to me that the "wild parties" were not as innocuous as she had originally described them, that they were, in fact, the setting for many episodes of sexual abuse Kira had experienced in her home. When she first began recounting the incidents, she did so with little apparent emotion. With each chilling account of the violations she had endured in her childhood, my desire to serve as a benign and protective presence in her life became more expansive. I was then a graduate intern, and Kira's life story was becoming my first "big" case of childhood sexual abuse. Guided by the language of "self as instrument," I had positioned myself to help her safely navigate the stages of recovery with textbook precision. To that end, I concentrated on helping her to name her experience, careful to shield her from the shame and self-doubt that was so much a part of her familial legacy.

As Kira talked more about herself, she recalled numerous episodes, each time reporting the details with a kind of detached wonder. For example, she casually mentioned learning how to sleep with screeching guitars as background "lullabies," or waking to find herself in the arms of a strange man, "probably a friend of my parents." She also mentioned the time one man mistook her bedroom for a bathroom and proceeded to urinate in her bed. In recalling the episodes, she described her father and mother more as errant adolescents than as abusive, neglectful parents. With each deadpan delivery of yet another horrific event, I came to see myself more and more as her champion–savior: the one who could help her not only see and come to terms with a painful past, but also begin to envision new ways of being in all of her relationships. For example, in the frequent conflicts with her boyfriend, Kira would quickly defer to his view of reality. She began to understand that in most instances, she had conceded to him the power to name. Therefore, if he described her as "moody," Kira's near-automatic response was to take on that description of herself as true. Kira and I began to use the language of "feeling-thoughts" (Miller, 1988) to help her give voice to her emotions, her needs, her angers, and her desires in, and her truths about, relationship. Over the course of the year, Kira asked me, many times, to bear witness to previously unnamed violations she had experienced during childhood. Once she brought in pictures of a party where she, at 6 years of age, sat on a man's lap, a friend of her parents whose name she could not recall ever knowing, and posed sucking his finger. At no time before our relationship had Kira thought of these encounters as abusive or even unusual. Having grown up in isolation as an only child in a substance-abusing family, the home environment provided her only template for normalcy.

Critical Junctures

A turning point in our therapy occurred when Kira recounted, with bemusement, her decision to run away from home when she was 9 years old. As we discussed it, there was nothing extraordinary about the decision itself. She was angry about not being allowed to go with her friends to a shopping mall. What was extraordinary was her plan to support herself when she struck out on her own. She had decided, quite matter-of-factly, that she could be a prostitute. Eleven years later she was incredulous that her career choice at the time had seemed as ordinary a choice as becoming a teacher or a pastry chef. With the articulation of this memory came fuller and deeper recall of other incidents, each more emotion laden than the one that preceded it. As I saw it, I was providing a safe harbor from which Kira could venture forth to explore the murky depths of a turbulent sea of childhood memories. With each session, she gained more courage to name and claim what she encountered in her explorations.

The naming of feelings and the associated thoughts helped her to clarify the vague unease she felt as a teenager, embarrassed to introduce her friends to her "hippie" parents. When I asked if there were specific fears associated with her unease, she responded that she never knew if her father might remove his swimming trunks, as he sometimes did with her when they were in their backyard pool. She also recalled a time when she and her mother were standing together at the kitchen sink, and her father came forward and fondled them both. In her mind, her mother's silent complicity legitimized the blatant violations by her father. Furthermore, the fact that she could recall no instance of genital penetration left her mistrustful of her own perceptions. With no one to witness her unease or to label the behavior as inappropriate, she accepted her father's interpretation of the abuse: that they were a close family. Moreover, her need for her parents' attention and her appreciation of her father's protectiveness nullified any claim that she might have for a different kind of togetherness.

Convinced, as I was, that Kira had been violated through years of parental neglect and sexual exploitation, it was relatively easy to concentrate on the past interpersonal/intrafamilial disconnections—disconnections *external* to our relationship—that had brought suffering into her life. That she had courageously survived years of what we agreed to term "low-grade trauma" in her family of origin was undeniable. Likewise, the effects of that trauma—silence, shame, and self-doubt—were equally obvious. It was relatively easy to focus on Kira's father and, in no small way, her mother as agents of traumatizing disconnection.

Over the course of a few months, Kira and I settled into an easy comfort with each other. We occasionally talked about one or another issue that came up as Kira worked on her senior thesis. One conversation went something like this:

KIRA: When I started working on this project, I realized how lucky am I to have the connections I got when I transferred to this school.

MAUREEN: I didn't realize you transferred here. Where did you go first?

KIRA: Oh, I started at [City University]. But my father made me transfer because he said it was too full of niggers and Puerto Ricans.

MAUREEN: (*without a pause*) And how was that decision for you? What did you want?

KIRA: Well, I knew that even though my father is a little bit prejudiced, he only wanted what was best for me. And he had a lot of confidence that I could be successful in a very good school.

I noticed but did not respond to the fact that Kira was smiling throughout this deadpan description of events. My response felt hollow, but it also felt like the best I could do. Indeed, I felt discomfort with this disclosure and wondered if it might be evidence of my imperfection as an "instrument" for her healing. Doubting the validity of my own feeling-thoughts, I was unable to bring them into relationship—either with Kira or with my supervisor.

Over the course of the year, as Kira developed more confidence in her perceptions, she grew increasingly able to tolerate her own feelings. Most of the time, however, she continued to talk about herself as someone who grew up with weird, neglectful, and perhaps sexually inappropriate parents, minimizing the impact of the chronic abuse. One day shortly before termination, Kira showed up at my office totally enraged. She was carrying a letter from her mother—a response to a letter Kira had written telling her mother about her longstanding sadness and anxiety, and demanding to know why she had not been more protected as a child. The mother, now divorced from the father, sent back a neatly typed letter conceding that (1) things probably got out of control during the party years, and (2) that therapy was nice but essentially useless, since worrying about the past would do no good. She ended the letter by admonishing Kira to be grateful for the experiences that helped her become a strong person and by asking if she was getting along better with her boyfriend. Kira sobbed deeply in that session, as I gave witness to the terrible isolation and unnamed hopelessness she had felt all her life. Over the final few weeks of our time together, Kira's gratitude was palpable. I knew that she trusted our relationship as a place where she would be heard and emotionally held.

Termination and Beyond

As she prepared for graduation, we began to terminate our relationship. In our final session, Kira was trying to explain the impact I had had on her life.

KIRA: I remember the first day I came to this office. It was hard for me to decide that I needed therapy, but I was feeling so bad most of the time. And I was afraid that Gary [her boyfriend] might leave me if I didn't get better.

MAUREEN: I'm glad you decided to come. It was such a big step for you.

KIRA: Yeah, then I remember seeing you walk down the stairs—and I saw that you were black! I just wanted to get up and run out of here. But I was desperate, and I wanted to be polite. I'm so glad I stayed and gave you a chance. When we got to your office, I was amazed at how well you spoke English and that you were saying some things that made sense to me. So I decided to come back, and by the third visit, I knew you were going to be good, and now it's hard for me to even think about being without you.

MAUREEN: [I was frankly blindsided by Kira's revelation and remained silent for what seemed like several moments before I was able to respond. I thought that in her painfully awkward way, Kira wanted to convey the depth of her gratitude. Aware of the 5 minutes we had left in our lives together, and wanting to remain empathic and authentic to the end, I mouthed the following statement.] It must have taken a lot of courage for you to risk revealing so much of yourself to someone whom you initially mistrusted.

One month later I received a letter from Kira, again expressing gratitude for the help she had received and informing me that she was getting along famously with her new therapist. She described him as a wonderful man, handsome like her father. With her new therapist, she had made some startling discoveries. First, she informed me, he had helped her to see that she was a victim of childhood sexual abuse and had, in fact, been a "surrogate spouse" to her father. Second, with the help of her new therapist, she was preparing to enter an inpatient program in a private hospital for the treatment of codependency.

My reaction was one of full-fledged ambivalence. On the one hand, it was gratifying to hear that Kira was continuing with her therapy, and that in fact, our work together had cleared a pathway toward further healing. On the other, I was saddened, angry, and feeling guilty. I was saddened that our work had ended for me on a note of discord and disconnection. Because I had rendered myself nearly invisible in my relationship with her (presumably for her "protection"), Kira had left the relationship quite happy—and quite oblivious of her impact on me. Indeed, upon receiving her letter, I felt as if I had been invisible: Kira's recent "discovery" of sexual abuse seemed to all but nullify the impact of our work together. I also felt guilty, wondering if my tentative and partial presence in our relationship may have hindered or slowed her tendency to trust her own perceptions. For example, I had exercised near unilateral control over the content of our sessions. When Kira ventured into territory that I deemed inappropriate, I exercised my privilege as therapist to determine what was appropriate and important to discuss. When she broached the topic of race, my response discouraged any examination of the images and distortions that impinged on our relationship. The images she brought into our relationship defined me as incompetent. Her letter seemed to indicate that she left the relationship not fully convinced otherwise. I, on the other hand, brought into the relationship images that generated anxiety about proving my competence both to my white client *and* my white supervisor. Perhaps because I had stifled Kira's efforts to speak her thoughts and examine her perceptions, she had had no recourse but to act them out. Finally, her apparent acceptance of her new therapist's diagnosis followed her learned pattern, once again, of conceding the power to name to an all-knowing authority figure. Although she had begun to resist her boyfriend's description of her as moody and her father's description of their family as close, she had now accepted her therapists' naming of her as codependent.

CASE ANALYSIS AND DISCUSSION

Perhaps two of the more useful questions that can be asked at this juncture are (1) what really happened in this relationship, and (2) how did it happen? That Kira was able to begin claiming her voice in her relationship with her parents and engaging her boyfriend with more confidence and clarity indicates some movement toward healing. However, those outcomes are attenuated, at best, in light of the dissonance that was apparent at the time of our termination. Throughout our relationship, I presented myself to Kira as the "perfect" instrument—an available and protective object, stripped of cultural context and emotional range. Because I had withheld vital parts of my experience from our relationship, Kira could not use our emergent process to expand her own relational capacities. It is no small wonder that in that final encounter, Kira might experience her gratitude for our relationship as an indication of her ability to tolerate our racial differences.

How did it happen that an otherwise "successful" therapy ended with a disempowering sense of disconnection between the therapist and the client? An exhaustive response is beyond the scope of this chapter, but even a brief analysis must begin with an examination of meta-assumptions: the cultural presumptions that guided the conduct of the therapeutic interventions. In the conduct of the interventions, there were no egregious departures from the norms of standard practice. Each intervention could be supported by some theoretical rationale/rationalization drawn from the culture of standard psychological practice. For example, I adopted a very supportive stance in my early conversations with Kira. Although I often noticed incongruence between her verbal content and her nonverbal behavior, I was initially focused on developing a level of rapport that would enable her to tell her story. Aware of the shame-infused nature of that story, I was very careful to avoid premature confrontation.

When Kira initially used racially inflamed language to describe her father's sentiments, I explained my lack of responsiveness to the content to myself as careful and caring attentiveness to process. Without a doubt, Kira's presenting issues required my most earnest and thoughtful interventions. However, the practice of relational–cultural therapy is not an either–or proposition. Earnest and thoughtful interventions that address a specific clinical issue need not preclude confronting the cultural power dynamics that shape the therapy relationship, as well as the presentation of the issue itself. Kira's remarks could reasonably be interpreted as resistance to the growing intimacy between us. The fact that our relationship involved perhaps her first close encounter with someone racially different from herself—someone imaged as her inferior—would no doubt elicit strategies of disconnection. Her remarks spoke directly to our relational context: a culture of misaligned, racially distorted power. Speaking directly to the issues that Kira raised might have signaled to her my willingness to walk with her through the minefields of racially charged conflict. My attempt to engage the clinical issues using a *presumptively* culture-blind framework impeded the development of empathy, authenticity, and mutuality in the relationship, the very healing processes so necessary to her growth.

In the relational–cultural model, disconnection is viewed as the primary source of human suffering (Jordan, 1997b). Although we most often think of disconnection or violation as an interpersonal, usually dyadic, event, it is also clear that the dominant culture itself may be the agent of wounding disconnection (Walker, 1999). Kira came into therapy with a very compelling issue that allowed me to ignore the complex relational distortions endemic to a racially stratified culture. These distortions manifest inevitably in relational images, feeling/thoughts that shape not only how people see themselves and interpret the meanings of past and current relationships, but also inform how they conceptualize relational possibilities (Miller & Stiver, 1997). Both Kira and I entered the relationship with "racialized biographies"—cultural histories that give rise to particular relational images. When such images go unaddressed, they flourish underground, thereby perpetuating the distortions that impede the flow of relational movement. Because of my unwillingness to bring these images explicitly and overtly into our relationship, our therapy became, in part, a reenactment of what Jordan (1997b) describes as societal traumatization: a social force that effectively silences people by moving them into self-doubt and shame.

Based on years of academic and clinical research, Janet Helms (1990) has also written convincingly about the impact of racial socialization on psychological functioning. In fact, she contends that any discussion of what we call personality is incomplete without an examination of racial identifications, irrespective of the racial group membership of the persons involved. Because racial identification is concerned with meaning making, the term is broadly compatible with what is called relational images in relational–cultural nomenclature. These images or identifications manifest in a variety of distorted power practices, many of which were enacted in my relationship with Kira. These distorted power practices might reasonably be termed strategies of disconnection. Exacerbating the effects of racial power-over practices were particular norms of standard clinical practice that function to cement the dominant–subordinate relationship between the therapist and client firmly in place. As was mentioned previously, most often these practices are meant to reinforce the boundaries of the relationship by securing power in the hands of the therapist, with the presumption that such an arrangement benefits the hapless client. This presumption is, in effect, a "trickle down" theory of power, which in therapy (as in economics) rarely supports the interests of the more vulnerable participant in the relationship.

In a racially stratified culture, as in any power-over culture, people are divided into dominant and subordinate, superior and inferior (Miller,

1976) Relational images, then, are also based on premises of "better than" and "less than." Although these racial belief systems (sometimes termed "internalized dominance" and "internalized oppression") trigger a variety of disconnection strategies, the shared behavioral and attitudinal theme is the dichotomization of power. The felt sense of vulnerability, inevitable under such arrangements, is answered with boundary protection, with an overemphasis on self-containment, autonomy, separateness, and control. Since the fundamental effect of the arrangement is to preserve the relational image and the power status quo, participants in these nonrelational arrangements remain unknown and unreal to themselves and to each other. An examination of our beginning sessions illustrates how racialized power distortions resulted in the enactment of therapeutically rationalized strategies of disconnection.

When Kira entered my office, I was aware, in principle, that I was about to enter a relationship with a young white woman who had been culturally indoctrinated to believe herself superior to me, a socialization rendered often more powerful for its subtlety. Likewise, as a matter of political principle, I was aware of the consistent if subtle socialization that would have me believe myself inferior to my white clients. I was less attuned to the actively mutating images deriving from that socialization. Nor was I aware of how a nonrelational framework might mask or exaggerate the resulting strategies of disconnection. In the therapy with Kira, two racialized strategies of disconnection were prominent. The first is what William Cross (1992) has termed "spotlight anxiety"; the second is what I like to call "racelessness."

When a relational encounter is defined by spotlight anxiety, excessive energy is channeled into managing the impressions of other people in a way that (1) supports one's vested image of self, and perhaps more important, (2) staves off the potential for disconnection. Committed, as I was, to the language of "self as instrument" instead of "relationship as pathway," I felt it was preeminently important to present a self that was highly competent and professionally informed. It was important *to me* to establish myself with Kira as one who could witness and bear her pain, and ultimately as one who could provide (as opposed to co-create) a relationship that could help her heal the ravages of abuse. In short, I needed Kira as a witness to my competence. This need was a survival strategy that was as much a product of the culture of therapy as of the culture of racism. The culture of clinical training demanded that therapists exhibit certainty, power, and invulnerability in their relationships with clients. Mindful that Kira may have been culturally indoctrinated to see me as incompetent, this strategy was as much an antidote to manage racial anxiety as it was an effort to comply with the norms and expectations of standard practice. Obviously, such a stance is opposed to the operation of empathy, authenticity, and mutuality in relationship. First, because I was unable to represent myself with clarity in the relationship, I was unable to access or sustain a connection with my own feeling-thoughts. While I concentrated great energy in demonstrating empathy toward Kira (or at least those parts of herself that I allowed her to bring into relationship), I was less empathic toward my own vulnerability. Accordingly, I could not represent that vulnerability with any sense of authenticity and intentionality in our relationship. Only those parts of myself that were likely to be affirmed or appreciated by Kira were allowed into the therapy room.

A strategy often employed to mitigate spotlight anxiety is racelessness. This strategy represents a usually conscious attempt to disconnect from one's cultural biography, especially a biography that is socially degraded. The belief underlying this strategy is that the extent to which one is viewed as an ahistorical being—a being without cultural context—is an indication of one's social worth or professional competence. (This belief is expressed in statements such as "I want to be seen as a great artist, not a great African/Chinese/Greek artist.") Ethnicity, particularly one that has been historically marginalized, is experienced as a source of limitation; one is enlarged by shedding it. Jenkins (1993) has alluded to this phenomenon in her work on the problem of social esteem. In many instances—and in this instance with Kira—racelessness as a strategy of disconnection is used to deny the personal and present implications of the political reality of racial inequality. Authenticity, as both goal and process, is essential to the unfolding of growth-enhancing movement. In other words, a marker of a healthy, healing relationship is one in which participants become increasingly able to represent themselves with clarity and accountability. My silence in response to Kira's invitation to address racial conflict was both an empathic failure and a failure of authenticity. As a result, both Kira and I missed an opportunity to move toward deeper connection. I not only stalled in my own development, I could not help Kira bring important aspects of her experience into our relationship. As Jordan (1997a) has eloquently noted, when the therapist can be empathic with her own experience—in this case, the experience of racial degradation—she can be more attuned to the whole fabric of the client's social and emotional world. To paraphrase Jordan, empathy across levels of stratified power begins with self-empathy. By developing empathy for our own racial/ethnic privileges and deprivations, our strengths and weaknesses, we transform disconnection into a source of connection.

Kira, for her part, was well practiced in strategies of disconnection stemming from internalized dominance. The most obvious are those that are based on what I call "secure disbelief in the Degraded Other." This relational image carries with it expectations of the Other's inferiority that range from benign surprise at the Other's demonstrated worth or competence to outright exclusion or rejection based primarily, or solely, on his or her degraded status. By her own report, Kira's disbelief in my competence triggered an impulse to exclude: She felt an urge to flee from the building rather than trust that an African American therapist could be helpful to her. Her impulse to exclude gradually shifted to surprise—first at my ability to "speak English" and later at her own experience of relief. In retrospect, it is obvious that the images deriving from sociopolitical inequality were in active interplay throughout the course of our relationship. The power of these images was such that we were compelled to enact that which we could not speak.

There was a powerful irony in that enactment. Partially to protect myself against the shame and vulnerability of social degradation, I adopted strategies of disconnection—which I could not have named as such at the time—that were guaranteed to fit perfectly with those Kira had been trained to enact. Patricia Hill Collins (1990) writes that one of the popular controlling images of African American women is that of the Mammy, the selfless, decontextualized servant who works endlessly and happily to satisfy the needs and whims of her superiors. The Mammy is presented as Superhuman in many respects, and in that rendering made subhuman, as she has no needs, no voice, no relational–cultural context other than that defined by her service to her superiors. By failing to address the relational images (i.e., our racialized biographies) at work in our relationship, I participated in the reenactment of a degraded, controlling image. By decontextualizing myself, I sought to appear controlled, masterful, unfailingly competent, and available. To the extent that I became raceless, our relationship became, in many respects, yet another variation on the superior–inferior theme so familiar in popular culture as the Mammy metaphor.

If the goal of therapy is to enlarge relational capacity—that is, to participate in relationship in increasingly complex ways—then it is imperative to relinquish old relational images. In other words, growing through action in relationship is a disruptive process. When the therapist and the client are able to move toward increasing authenticity, old images derived from past relationship and from the larger culture are rearticulated or otherwise released. In my relationship with Kira, large parts of my experience were withheld from the relationship (presumably for Kira's good). Therefore, Kira's relational images—the meanings and expectations she ascribed to racial difference—remained largely intact.

No analysis would be complete without exploring how the culture of therapy itself may reproduce and exacerbate the impact of cultural stratification. Linda James Meyers (1988) has written that overemphasis on material reality results in a suboptimal psychology. The characteristic ontological stance of such a psychology is one that values extreme individualism as well as the acquisition and control of resources. Because such resources are invariably seen as limited, the inevitable result is social paranoia. This worldview that Meyers describes is implicated in the therapeutic quest for the atomized, independent self, a bounded entity capable of exercising mastery and control over impulses and social and material resources (Jordan, 2002). The implications are clear: When containment, separation, and control are the dominant goals of social behavior, all relationships are infused with some degree of zero-sum competition or the dichotomization of power. Likewise, underneath each relational encounter lies the subterranean goal of establishing power over, or winning. Each relational encounter, including therapy, is an event to be won. Strategies of disconnection, deployed by both therapist and client, provide the illusion of winning—either by establishing power over or forestalling the threat of being overpowered.

My response to Kira's racially charged remarks nicely illustrates this point. When Kira announced her father's prejudice against "niggers and Puerto Ricans," I could not fail to notice the provocative intent of her statement, particularly as it was underscored by her tacit agreement with his assessment ("He's a bit prejudiced, but wants what's best for me . . . "). I was, in fact, unsettled by what I experienced as her "more than a little smug" presentation. From my vantage point as therapist, however, I exercised the privilege of making a unilateral determination that *Kira* was not ready to delve into such charged material, particularly as it might distract her from more urgent therapeutic goals. As I mentioned earlier, I also entertained the notion that she introduced off-putting material as a resistance strategy. With these interpretations that located the client as the sole repository of vulnerability, I was able to effectively deny my own trepidation. I also spoke in supervision about the importance of timing as a strategy for *winning* Kira's trust. Few of us would question the centrality of trust in the therapeutic relationship. However, in a power-over paradigm, trust is construed as a something of a commodity, the proper distribution of which involves an upward flow, from client to therapist. Nowhere in this meta-assumption is there a metaphor for defining trust as an ebb and flow between client and therapist in the process of building faith in the relationship. Although all of the interpretations were plausible, they begged the question of mutual trust. My conscious intent was to respond to Kira in a way that would allow her to trust me, that would show her that I would neither judge nor abandon her for her or her parents' racial beliefs. However, I did not allow her to explore those beliefs and images in relationship with me. It occurred to me in that session that perhaps Kira wanted us to talk about our relationship. Indeed, under other circumstances—perhaps with a same-race client, perhaps with less inflamed language—I would have pursued the opportunity to explore living, in-the-moment, process. I remember, however, making the decisions not to put *Kira* "on the spot" (or spotlight) and risk making *her* uncomfortable so early in our relationship. Kira, in effect, presented an invitation into a new level of anxiety and conflict, one that would bring us into more present connection with each other.

It is also worth noting that shame about what I viewed as my own emotional weakness belied my dogged attempts to win Kira's trust. As a fledging clinical trainee, I was fearful of feeling hurt or angered by Kira's use of a racial slur; such an emotional reaction might signal my unfitness to be a therapist. Implicit in my thinking was the notion that I should have been strong enough to remain unfazed by Kira's revelation; that perhaps, if only to myself, I should have been able to construct an interpretation that would allow me to feel less vulnerable. The idealized images that I held cast the therapist as the perfect "self as instrument." This perfect therapist could and should withstand any onslaught, no matter how meanspirited or virulent it might be. Secure in her expertise (e.g., creative insights, perfectly crafted interpretations), my ideal inner therapist could and should remain purposeful and controlled, in full mastery of the moment. In other words, the ideal therapist was the ultimate embodiment of the traditional notions of the fully individuated, autonomous Healthy Self. In the absence of explicit training and support to suggest otherwise, this power-over version of the Healthy Self becomes the default norm. The rigidity of this norm is such that emotional *avoidance* becomes the stand-in for emotional *resilience*. Interestingly, in the culture of therapy, I was in a low power position as an expendable psychology trainee. In the room with Kira, however, I could use the relatively more privileged position as helper/clinician to avoid confronting the present and historical pain that presented itself to me for healing.

From the perspective of the relational–cultural model, this avoidance represented a failure of mutuality. As noted in previous chapters, mutuality does not denote sameness. It does denote openness to influence. Unlike the impervious, impermeably boundaried therapist of the power-over model—the ideal therapist of my early imagination—the therapist who practices mutuality allows him- or herself to be influenced and emotionally moved by her client. Furthermore, the mutual empathy that develops in the relationship is such that the therapist is able to show his or her client that he or she has been moved (Jordan, 2003). As Miller has frequently noted, people experience wounding disconnection when they are unable to have an impact, or when they are unable to discern their impact, on others. To withhold relational information is to impede learning through action in relationship and to further deepen the wounds of disconnection.

Perhaps the poet Audre Lorde says it best. In a letter to her therapist, Lorde wrote:

This territory between us is new and frightening as well as urgent, rigged with pieces of our own individual racial histories which neither of us chose, but each of us bears the scars from. And those are particular to each of us. But there is a history we share because we are black women living in a racist sexist cauldron, and that means that some part of my journey is yours too. (1984, p. 162)

To practice mutuality is to recognize that although the client and therapist are not walking the *same* journey, they are on a *shared* journey. Walking a piece of the way with Kira would have allowed me to examine not just her readiness but my own willingness to navigate through the rigged racial histories that had left us both wounded, vulnerable, and enraged.

NARRATIVE REDUX

Our rigged histories of power-over stratification function to silence and shame anyone who risks engaging a relationship for the express purpose of promoting growth-enhancing change. Moreover, this shame is amplified by the meta-assumptions of unilateral control and dichotomous process characteristic of the power-over therapeutic frameworks.

Dichotomous process demands a yes/no, either/or response. It is a demand that stifles creativity. In my relationship with Kira, my stilted response to her admittedly provocative comments illustrates the constraints imposed by dichotomous process. The thinking probably went like this: "If I listen with respect and openness to her process, I may become angry and abandon Kira. Or, to listen with respect and openness to Kira may be to disrespect and abandon myself. Better to stay in control and focus on something she can handle." Thus followed safe, plausible interpretations and movement into territory that Kira's *therapist* could handle, secure in the illusion of power and control.

How might the conversation about the school transfer have gone differently? There is no perfect answer, no way to determine the outcome unilaterally. However, there are responses that would have been more expressive of my curiosity, more consistent with my intuitions, and more respectful of the emotional process that was forming between us.

KIRA: My father wanted me to transfer because he thought the school was too full of niggers and Puerto Ricans.

MAUREEN: [any of the following] How did you feel about the school? What was it like having that discussion with him? What is it like having that discussion with me? What do you think it is about blacks and Puerto

Ricans that's so offensive or dangerous? Those judgments are always hard for me to hear. I'd like for us to talk about how it feels for us to discuss them.

Although there is no perfect response, it is probably the case that any one of the above possibilities would have facilitated movement beyond the images into more enlivened relationship with each other. By representing myself more fully in relationship, I would have given Kira permission to do the same. To paraphrase Irene Stiver: when the therapist disconnects from her own experience and makes it unavailable to the relationship, the client is not free to represent herself with authenticity (Stiver, 1992). Again, the profound irony of the situation is that by focusing on winning her trust by withholding parts of myself from relationship, I may have inadvertently shamed parts of Kira out of relationship.

An often repeated maxim among relational–cultural practitioners is Stiver's advice to learn to say "one true thing" when faced with a confounding therapeutic dilemma. Again, in my final conversation with Kira, there were many true things to say, of which I might have selected one.

KIRA: Then I remember seeing you walk down the stairs—and I saw that you were black! I just wanted to get up and run out of here. But I was desperate and I wanted to be polite. I'm so glad I stayed and gave you a chance. When we got to your office, I was amazed at how well you spoke English and that you were saying some things that made sense to me. So I decided to come back, and by the third visit, I knew you were going to be good, and now it's hard for me to even think about being without you.

MAUREEN: I am always sad when people doubt my abilities because of race, and I can appreciate how difficult it must have been for you to share your story with someone you initially mistrusted.

I like to think (in retrospect and with benefit of many more years of experience) that a more authentic conversation might have fostered greater clarity in the connection between Kira and me, and ultimately may have allowed her to enter into a relationship with another therapist with a sense of her own competence and intentionality. Authentic responsiveness is not full disclosure. It is a process of attunement and accountability. It suggests movement into fuller and deeper connection with the feeling-thoughts of the moment and using clinical judgment to represent those thoughts that are potentially growth promoting in the relationship. What I felt most acutely at the time of our last conversation was profound fatigue, a sense of a never-ending struggle of living in a culture where blackness connotes inferiority or incompetence until proven otherwise. If there were words for that feeling, they would have expressed a sad resignation that "this will never end." There I was: armored, as it were, with excellent training, working in an elite institution, supported by nationally respected supervisors, and none of it was sufficient to protect me from the pain of the dominant culture—the shame and the anger of a racially stratified relationship. Not all of those thoughts would have been helpful in that particular relationship, and to fully disclose them at that time would be to risk fostering an environment of shaming reactivity. To fully withhold them meant that I would risk perpetuating ignorance and isolation.

Many years have passed since my encounter with Kira, yet our relationship continues to teach me the importance of accepting the invitation to walk a piece of the way with my clients. Interestingly, in African American culture, the practice of walking a piece of the way grew out of conditions of material vulnerability, commonly practiced among people who lacked ready access to automobiles. To walk a piece of the way in therapy is to acknowledge that any therapy, irrespective of apparent differences or similarities between client and therapist, is a cross-cultural journey fraught with shifting vulnerabilities. It is worth noting that power distortions associated with stratification are not confined to cross-racial relationships or to racial marginalization. In fact, it is important for white therapists and white clients to explore the silent assumptions of racial dominance and the impact of those assumptions on their relationship with each other as well as on their functioning in the larger world. It is important to explore those assumptions because the disconnections that surface in bold relief in cross-racial encounters often exist in muted form in the relational images and meanings that shape same-race relationships. In other words, social stratification gives rise to distorted images that constrain the relational development of both the dominant and marginalized group members. The disconnections created by politics of social stratification have a profound impact on psychological development and manifest in relationship, including those that exist for the express purpose of fostering clarity, healing, and connection.

The politics of stratification, of power over, is transformed into power *with* when client and therapist can risk exploring the meanings and images associated with race/ethnicity, sexuality, economic and social class, gender, or any of the socially salient markers that stratify the dominant culture. Working with Kira taught me that the path to connection is co-created by walking together through conflict—that which is a part of our cultural heritage, as well as that which inevitably arises in any relational endeavor. To navigate the shared journey is to embrace the differences, believing that, when represented with authenticity in relationship, differences are potential wellsprings of growth. Walking a piece of the way requires the therapist to assume responsibility for the power he or she holds in relationship, to respect the power his or her client holds, and to support the fluid interplay of influence. It is, in fact, an abuse of power to pretend to sameness (i.e., avoid conflict) and to preempt the growth-inducing possibilities that connecting across difference can bring. In the relational–cultural model, the therapist accepts responsibility for engaging the complexity of empathy, the vulnerability of authenticity, and the nuances of mutuality. He or she accepts responsibility for learning to walk a piece of the way.

REFERENCES

Collins, P. H. (1990). *Black feminist thought: Knowledge, consciousness, and the politics of empowerment*. Boston: Unwin Hyman.

Cross, W. E. (1992). *Shades of black: Diversity in African-American identity*. Philadelphia: Temple University Press.

Helms, J. E. (1990). *Black and white racial identity: Theory, research and practice*. Westport, CT: Praeger.

Jenkins, Y. (1993). Diversity and social esteem. In V. De La Cancela, J. Chin, & Y. Jenkins (Eds.), *Diversity in psychotherapy: The politics of race, ethnicity, and gender* (pp. 45–64). Westport, CT: Praeger.

Jordan, J. V. (1997a). Relational development through mutual empathy. In A. C. Bohart & L. S. Greenberg (Eds.), *Empathy reconsidered: New directions in psychotherapy* (pp. 343–351). Washington, DC: American Psychological Association.

Jordan, J. V. (1997b). Relational therapy in a non-relational world. *Work in Progress, No. 79*. Wellesley, MA: Stone Center Working Paper Series.

Jordan, J. V. (2002). Learning at the margin: New models of strength. *Work in Progress, No. 98*. Wellesley, MA: Stone Center Working Paper Series.

Jordan, J. V. (2003). Growth in connection. In L. Slater, J. H. Daniels, & A. Banks (Eds.), *The complete guide to women's mental health*. Boston: Beacon Press.

Lorde, A. (1984). *Sister outsider: Essays and speeches*. Freedom, CA: Crossing Press.

Meyers, L. J. (1988). *Understanding an Afrocentric world view: Introduction to an optimal psychology*. Dubuque, IA: Kendall/Hunt.

Miller, J. B. (1976). *Toward a new psychology of women*. Boston: Beacon Press.

Miller, J. B., & Stiver, I. P. (1997). *The healing connection: How women form relationships in therapy and in life*. Boston: Beacon Press.

Stiver, I. P. (1992). A relational approach to therapeutic impasses. *Work in Progress, No. 58*. Wellesley, MA: Stone Center Working Paper Series.

Walker, M. (1999). Race, self, and society: Relational challenges in a culture of disconnection. *Work in Progress, No. 85*. Wellesley, MA: Stone Center Working Paper Series.

4

Making Great Memories
Empathy, Derailment, and Growth

WENDY B. ROSEN

> The most helpful part of working with you is you don't keep
> yourself hidden. You talk about your family and your
> feelings. You've taught me that joy comes from the
> connection you have with others. Real connection, not just
> talking about connection. You've shown me that being
> vulnerable is not a liability but an asset to having healthy
> and honest relationships. I appreciate your wisdom to know
> when to work outside the box.
> —EXCERPT OF A LETTER FROM MAURA (A CLIENT)

THE THERAPEUTIC CONTEXT

Psychotherapy, at its heart, is all about relationship. The client comes to
the relationship with emotional injuries from earlier relational experiences and is seeking to be met in this place. Empathy, as defined by
relational–cultural theory, occupies a place of central importance in the
work of psychotherapy and is seen as fundamental to the healing process
(Jordan, Surrey, & Kaplan, 1981). Recovery from relational damage relies
strongly on the capacity of another to bear affective witness to earlier
wounds, and in so doing, to introduce a potentially new relational outcome in the present. Mutual empathy, or the capacity to be moved and to
feel the other being moved in concert, is of primary significance in gener-
ating alternative, growth-promoting experiences of relationship (Jordan,

1985). The fluid movement of such relationships carries its own poetry that stays with each person as relational image guiding future expectations and actions. These relational images accumulate over time and form a personal frame of reference for what relationships require for their maintenance. Not all relationships achieve moments of harmonious meeting, nor does any relationship experience them all the time. A growth-fostering relationship, however, is one that can move in and out of such meaningful moments of shared affective resonance with resilience, emerging with greater depth and breadth each time.

Given the paradox of connection—the longing for, yet terror of, connection—people tend to stay in relationship by keeping parts of themselves out of relationship, usually the most vulnerable parts (Miller & Stiver, 1997). As a result, moments of emotional contact between client and therapist can sometimes be quite complicated and conflicted. These moments offer essential experiences in therapy, however, if healing is to take place on injured, and thus more vulnerable, ground. Jean Baker Miller refers to the therapeutic aim of "waging good conflict" at these wounded places as a means of promoting mutual emotional and relational growth, as opposed to producing a winner and a loser. Good conflict, by definition, is one in which the aim is that of shared and broadened understanding, rather than the defeat of one over the other. A central component of this dynamic is the fact that client and therapist both come to these places of shared empathic potential with their own relational histories and derivative relational images (Rosen, 1999). Inevitably, there are times when injury touches injury, and these are the very moments that can be either mutually transformational or irreparably destructive. Some of the most profound points of contact occur at the boundary of the relationship, or "the intimate edge" (Ehrenberg, 1974).

In this therapeutic work, meeting in vulnerability, a state of accessible emotional openness and receptivity, is seen as a sign of strength, a window of possibility, and an essential precursor to the process of growth. It also speaks to the necessary nature of boundary permeability if a relationship is to move and expand into greater levels of resiliency. Although the primary focus in therapy is always the relational growth of the client, real therapeutic change, from a relational perspective, inevitably involves shared movement and expansion. Both client and therapist participate together in the bearing and authentic examination of what are sometimes painful moments of personal truth (Hartling, Rosen, Walker, & Jordan, 2000). The conduct of such an examination, particularly in terms of what is openly shared between client and therapist, bears a certain personal stamp that is unique to the relationship under scrutiny. Relational–cultural theory and professional ethics, however, must be in place as essential guideposts.

My earliest training as a clinician took place in the context of a traditional psychoanalytic theory and therapeutic protocol. Over time, however, the fundamental rules of engagement prescribed for the therapy relationship seemed to run counter to many of the therapeutic aims. In my experience, the psychoanalytic framework, at times, contributed to an interpersonal distance between client and therapist and a reliance more on the cognitive/intellectual aspects than the emotional, relational dynamic. Although interpretive understanding can certainly serve an important informative function in therapy, it alone fails to generate the necessary affective conditions for empathic exchange and emotional growth. Both thoughts and feelings, or as Jean Baker Miller has termed them, "feeling-thoughts," seemed to me to create a more comprehensive bridge connecting client and therapist. In addition, the more traditionally defined roles of therapist and "patient" seemed to be a potential breeding ground for an abuse of power on the part of the therapist. Although there are certain imbalances of power inherent in any "helping" relationship, the rigid distinction between the "expert" therapist and the "fragile" patient belies the complexity of this meeting of heart and mind and contains the seeds of potential rewounding via repetition of earlier relational injuries. In relational–cultural theory, healthy relationships are seen as resting resiliently on a fluidity of emotional expertise, experienced vulnerability and observational capacities, and the ability to acknowledge and bear this complexity in a context of "power with" versus "power over." It is the therapist's fundamental commitment and his or her professional ability to name and to bring some consistent, examined clarity to this complex emotional exchange that, among other things, distinguishes the role of therapist. These are the points of therapeutic encounter that have the power to contribute to, rather than arrest, mutual relational growth.

The case of Maura, discussed next, centers on just such an interaction. Maura's and my shared participation was emotionally challenging, inevitable, and mutually clarifying. In particular, this case demonstrates the idiosyncratic nature of every therapy relationship in terms of the two people involved. In other words, in any therapeutic relationship the work must be viewed in the context of the particular people at the particular time, including the interaction of relational images, cultural contexts, historical contributions, and current personal realities.

THE CASE OF MAURA

Setting the Stage

Some years before Maura entered individual therapy with me, I had worked with her and her partner in couple therapy. Maura was in a lesbian relationship, and the couple was referred to me in their request for a lesbian therapist with several years of experience. Their therapy took place for less than a year, culminating with Maura and her partner going their separate ways. In the short time that I had known Maura, I had witnessed a great deal about certain aspects of her relational strengths and challenges. I had felt very moved by her visible pain at the ending of the relationship, but was also struck by her no-nonsense approach to taking quick action and "moving on."

Quite some time later, Maura called to make an appointment for herself. She was in the midst of making an unexpected and critical decision that would clearly change her life and wanted my advice. One of Maura's sisters was in serious difficulty and could no longer responsibly care for her young daughter. Maura was considering taking over the raising of this child. We met once, and she eventually decided to proceed with guardianship. A few months later, I inadvertently heard through the grapevine within the lesbian community (a not-uncommon occurrence within a relatively small, minority population) that Maura's other sister had died quite suddenly. From my earlier work with her, I knew this was a particularly tragic loss that very likely would exceed her standard attempts to cope. The mode of excessive privacy and self-sufficiency was one of Maura's familiar strategies of disconnection. It was based on relational images about what she could expect from others (I will say more at a later point). Given the brief, but clearly significant, connection we had made, as evidenced by her uncharacteristic decision to call me about her niece, I made my own decision to reach out and call her to express my sorrow and extend my condolences. Although this unsolicited action certainly challenged the standards of therapeutic protocol in which I had earlier been trained, I based my decision on my existing relational experience with Maura, which, in my perception, warranted the unorthodox action. It was an effort to meet her own uncharacteristic action of calling me earlier. It was also a response to my felt awareness of what she might need. A willingness to "go the extra mile" for her was a way to speak to her own very apparent generosity of spirit, as well to a vast chasm of personal deprivation in this regard. She admitted being surprised but grateful to hear from me and readily acknowledged having an extremely difficult time emotionally. I reminded her that if things began to feel too unbearable on her own, she could consider therapy as a resource for herself, and I would gladly provide her with referral names. Maura said she would consider it at a later date, if she felt the need. A few months later Maura called me, after already having met with a few different therapists, and asked if she might meet with me for individual therapy.

What Maura Brought to the Therapy Relationship

Maura had grown up in a large first-generation Irish Catholic family with a history of extreme poverty on both sides. Maura's mother was often

quite stressed and took out her frustrations, both emotionally and physically, on Maura as the eldest of several children. Maura was perceived as
the "tough one" who could take and handle anything and needed very little. Although Maura has always resented her mother for this treatment,
she also perceived her as a survivor and admired her accomplishments.
Her father, whom she had always idolized, taught her early on that she
would have to be strong throughout her life, and particularly that she
would have to fight her own battles, both literally and figuratively.
Maura's father was always an ardent and vocal proponent of the importance of family bonds. Yet one day during Maura's teenage years, he suddenly left, abandoning the family with no notice. This left Maura feeling
stunned, betrayed, angry, and enormously responsible for the welfare of
her siblings. She has since taken care of each of them at various times in
her life and in multiple ways, often providing shelter and money.

Maura grew up to become a successful businesswoman whose philosophy is captured in a quote she shared with me that hangs over her desk.
It reads

> Every morning in Africa, a gazelle wakes up. It knows it must run faster
> than the fastest lion or it will be killed. Every morning in Africa, a lion
> wakes up. It knows it must run faster than the slowest gazelle or it will
> starve. It doesn't matter whether you are a lion or a gazelle—when the sun
> comes up, you'd better be running.

Maura's family history, cultural background, and quoted philosophy
say a great deal about her current relational images. In her experience,
life is a constant fight-or-flee struggle for survival in a dangerous, unpredictable, and competitive environment. She has learned that in order to
have relationships, she must be perceived as strong and invulnerable, rendering invisible her own fragile feelings and needs. Past experience has
proven to her that important others will shame or abandon her, in one
way or another, if she demonstrates feelings and needs. Maura has
learned to speak the language of action and deed, and much less so, the
language of feeling. She perceives emotional dependency as entirely too
subject to abuse, betrayal, and loss. Being generously given to is not part
of her experience in life. Early on in therapy she emphasized the point
that "I will never want what I cannot have." In other words, Maura's central relational paradox is to maintain relationships by keeping her feelings, wants, and needs—what she perceives as the more wounded and
vulnerable parts of herself—out of the relationship. The one person in her
life who came closest to knowing this more hidden side of Maura was the
sister closest in age to her, her best friend, the one whose sudden death
occasioned my call.

Maura is an extraordinarily generous person; she readily gives of herself to others whenever she perceives a need. She invests time and energy, as well as material goods, without expectation of reciprocity. In her gift giving for every important occasion, she is remarkably precise and thoughtful. Her generosity, as she defines it, "is not about anything. It is who I am." On the one hand, this is one of many appealing characteristics that Maura brings to a relationship, and in some ways, an important source of personal worth and empowerment. On the other hand, her generosity can paradoxically serve as a strategy of disconnection at times. Maura's immense generosity can function to mask or offset her own underlying needs for such precision care, primarily emotionally, but also in the form of a helping hand. It also keeps her from knowing and trusting the full range and power of her capacity to be generous on an emotional level, as well as knowing her own value to others beyond what she has to give them. By inadvertently "protecting" herself in this way, she effectively maintains a certain relational distance and thus preempts the feared possibility of shame, disappointment, or loss.

On the other hand, Maura can also be quite exacting when it comes to "doing your job." As a manager/boss, she is very concerned about the welfare of her employees, but she also holds high standards and expectations of performance. At times, she feels personally hurt by any semblance of failure on their part. This holds true, as well, in her relationship with her niece, regarding particular household and personal responsibilities. Maura has a powerful voice—one she trusts and uses articulately—when she feels certain of her convictions. She is, however, quite capable of precipitously flying off the handle in a daunting manner when she feels she has been treated disrespectfully. In fact, she has been known to completely sever a relationship in the face of such perceived disrespect. When she feels personally disregarded and hurt, her outbursts of anger can become another strategy of disconnection. To fight for what she wants and to flee in the face of dangerous disappointment have been strong, characteristically defining modes in Maura's relational experiences and expectations.

WHAT I BROUGHT TO THE THERAPY RELATIONSHIP

I grew up in an Eastern European Jewish family with a history of anti-Semitic persecution on both sides. This legacy has left intergenerational threads of fear, mistrust, and quiet self-deprecation in its wake. Both of my parents grew up during the Depression in households that felt keenly the effects of both these influences, and thus, the ensuing tensions and challenges to a sense of self-worth. Neither of my parents' families knew much restraint when it came to heated temperaments and punishing outbursts, and this volatility carried over into my family, as well. This larger cultural as well as familial context has contributed to my current relational images and strategies of disconnection. Growing up Jewish, and later, coming out as a lesbian have meant living with forces that counter my sense of personal and relational value. These include both real and imagined threats to my overall safety and integrity. This history has left me with the perception that fundamental realities of my personal identity are subject to being shamed and disdained, and thus, if they become known, my relationships with these individuals will become threatened in some way. Overcompensation in other areas has served me as a means not only of managing this fear but also as a strategy of disconnection, lest my inner sense of unworthiness be discovered.

My relationship with my father has also served as a challenge. My father is an ideologically conservative, easily threatened, big-tempered, yet privately very tender man. He has taught me much about mistrusting one's own perceptions and integrity. A very intelligent man, but prone to feeling unduly challenged and shamed, he has been both the Wizard of Oz and the man behind the curtain. In my relationship with him, I have learned the necessity of searching behind and beneath to find him, but also to keep silent about what I see. Acting on my sensitivity to his hidden realities of tenderness and injury felt necessary to establishing a real connection with him. He perceives the overt acknowledgment of such relationally valuable knowledge, however, as being shamefully exposed in his vulnerability, and his typical response is some form of angry disconnection.

Silence, or alternatively, speaking in a voice not my own, have therefore become my own familiar strategies of disconnection in paradoxical efforts at engagement.

MEETING IN MUTUAL VULNERABILITY

Maura gave me gifts on occasion, each one quite thoughtful. Although I accepted them, I was somewhat reticent because I did not want her to feel that gift giving was the price of either my caring or valuing of her. Neither did I want her to feel challenged and shamed in her gestures of generosity. It felt like a delicate balance between overtly valuing her very real generosity and self-worth as a giver, while honoring her strategies of disconnection from the complex of feelings upon which such giving may have also rested. More than once, I shared my reticence with her. Each time, she countered with a suggestion of moderate frustration, telling me that I have always "gone the extra mile" for her whenever she needed me, and how much she has appreciated my generosity. For me, any evidence of Maura's increasing sense of emotional freedom and competence and the strengthening of her convictions about her worthiness to be loved was the most valuable "gift" I could ever receive from her. She, however, could not yet know or believe this. The complexity of feelings around giving and receiving and worthiness were not limited to Maura alone. I, too, carried complicated relational images that made it quite difficult for me, on some level, to feel worthy of being valued for my "gifts" of understanding, empathy, and good care, and being responded to in kind. I, too, had strategies of disconnection in the face of fearing challenges to my sense of self-worth or being seen as a vulnerable, and thus incompetent, caregiver. Although I believed in my capacities and integrity as a therapist, through years of experience, at the same time, a lifetime of experiencing fundamental challenges to my personal identity still served as a magnet for uncertainty.

During the course of our therapy, I had given Maura a couple of small gifts for no special reason, except that they reminded me of her and significant points in our work together. In some ways, I felt they served as concrete representations of certain empathic connections, a kind of visible punctuation mark in the therapy relationship. In response, Maura was appreciative, although somewhat reserved, in her response. At times, her response bordered on an almost imperceptible but nonetheless awkward discomfort. I chose not to address the feeling, since it appeared to me at the time to serve as perhaps a necessary strategy of disconnection in the face of feeling vulnerable. Rather than challenge it, I honored it until all of what was at play began to feel clearer. Only later, after Maura and I had gone through a painful but transformational process of relational disconnection and repair, did I learn to reexamine my working perspective.

At Christmas one year, I gave Maura a present to give to her niece, Cara. My conscious motivation at the time involved feeling deeply touched by Maura's immense generosity of spirit and her devoted commitment to raising her niece, despite the personal compromises this entailed. She often described her many activities with Cara and her little friends as acts of "making great memories." In giving a gift for Cara, I hoped to acknowledge some of Maura's most loving relational "work" to date in her creation of a family. When I gave it to Maura, I found myself feeling curiously awkward and downplaying the gift, saying it was just "a little thing" for her niece, "no big deal," "just a little something." In point of fact, it was not at all an elaborate gift, but it was a meaningful gesture nonetheless. In retrospect, I could see that my own relational paradox had come into play. I believe I was attempting to protect myself by preempting Maura's typically lukewarm response to a gift. Although the gift itself reflected something touching and valuable that I perceived in her, my manner was apologetic, self-conscious, and focused on the quality of the gift.

My own relational images of giving, of feeling not very valued for what I had to give, and the relative worth of my gifts, per se, were clearly driving the discomfort of my actions and obstructing my attempt at conveying the real message of how moved I was by her. In my own history, acts of giving were ambivalent and value-laden affairs. I was interacting with Maura as if I would be judged or criticized by her. Maura's response was a bit hesitant, including some nervous laughter at my uncomfortable verbal fumbling. Neither of us addressed this interplay of feeling, rendering us rather disconnected while we quickly moved on to other subjects. Both of us allowed and sustained this disconnection for the remainder of the hour. Maura could not address my vulnerability, lest she wound and potentially lose me. I could not address Maura's nonchalance in her receipt of the gift, lest I challenge her vulnerability and strategy of disconnection in the face of being given to. By failing to meet and connect in our mutually felt vulnerability, we generated a rupture that would lead to a ripple effect preceding our efforts at repair.

At our next session, I found myself feeling irrationally hurt that I had received no feedback from Maura about the gift. Maura, too, seemed to carry an air of reticence about her that typically appeared when there was something uncomfortable on her mind. She had barely sat down in her chair when I impulsively asked her what Cara had thought of the gift. She shifted uncomfortably and said to me, "Well, we opened it, and what I want to know is whether somebody gave that to you, and you didn't want it, so you handed it down to us." I felt stunned and shamefully accused, responding with an immediate and firm denial to her question. She accepted this response, and once again, we moved on in mutually feigned connection discussing nothing that either of us could remember. I remained very upset about this interaction throughout the remainder of the day, and while I had some loosely connected thoughts about it, I knew I needed help in understanding what had happened to cause this rupture in our relationship. I therefore turned to a trusted colleague for consultation, rather than attempt to figure this out in shamed isolation.

The consultation proved to be extremely helpful. My colleague was able to empathize with my experience of hurt and shame, rather than condemn me for having "unprofessional" feelings. She also helped me to step back from the experience and reclaim my observing capacities. From this vantage point, I became able to look at the feelings as part of a continuously moving set of relational interactions between Maura and me, rather than as a static and isolated lapse in the treatment. Together, my colleague and I were able to play with tentative observations on the possible mutual contributions to this "moment" in the therapy relationship. Those contributions were shaped by some of the more complicated relational images around giving that both Maura and I brought to our relational dynamic.

The consultation with my colleague, which was both empathic and educational, became an important healing relational experience in and of itself, one that enabled me to hold onto my relationship with Maura and bear the painful uncertainty of our temporary breach.

At our next session, I told Maura that I thought we needed to talk about what had happened between us in the preceding appointment. I offered that I had had a wounded reaction to her accusation about the gift and that I had pulled away during our session. Maura responded, "God! You're so sensitive!" She agreed that she had felt my distance, but she had not related it to her comment. She imagined that I had other personal things on my mind and that maybe I had not felt like meeting that day. Maura felt she could not ask me about it at the time, since it was very likely my "personal business." I confirmed for Maura that, in fact, I am sensitive, which is both good and difficult sometimes. I suggested to her that perhaps both of our sensitivities met up in the last session and were touched by what it means to give and to be given to. While I had felt hurt by her comment about my gift, I acknowledged that my own complicated personal issues about value and worth had fed my response and fueled my disconnection from her, as I had felt ashamed. I proposed to Maura that her comment might have revealed something about her feelings that had to do with her family background of extreme poverty. Perhaps an old relational image for her was one of gifts from others in the sole form of hand-me-downs, and thus expressive of no feeling from the giver other than pity. In a culture that denigrates poverty, shame often replaces gratitude and puts the person in a disconnecting fight mode. She agreed that she had felt deflated at the notion that the gift might have been a discarded hand-me-down, and she had "just wanted to check it out." I told Maura that I had felt troubled by our mutual detachment and that I had sought consultation in order to try and figure out what had happened. I said it had helped me to come back in an effort to examine the rupture and figure out a way to repair it with her. Maura was struck by how strongly I had felt about the interaction and that I would make an effort to talk it over with someone. Coming back to her in an effort to examine the breach together and then to mutually learn and grow from it formed a new set of relational images for each of us in different ways. Rather than permanently retreating from conflict in shame or fear, our history together thus far allowed us to test whether the relationship could handle efforts at repair. We were able to begin the work of waging good conflict.

Maura began the next session by reading to me a list of responses she had felt from our last discussion. As becomes clear, she felt able to express some of her more powerful feelings about our interaction. The list consisted of the following responses:

1. "I thought it was safe to talk. I didn't think about your feelings."
2. "I never even had my coat off before you asked about the gift."
3. "Yes, I'm a little slow at expressing emotions, but whose time clock do I need to be on?"
4. "You set me up by minimizing and devaluing gifts you give me."
5. "You disconnected from me during our session, and it says on page 32 or something of that book you gave me [*The Healing Connection*] that that's not a good thing."
6. "What hurts me the most is that you didn't talk to me first about your feelings, that you didn't trust me enough and had to go to someone else instead."

The clarity of Maura's feelings was potent and came from a very authentic place within her. Her observations could find no argument from me, nor did I experience shame in her accurate perception of my behavior. Rather, I felt moved by Maura's trust of our relationship to both come back in the middle of our conflict and to speak her truth to me. There existed a flow of mutual empathy between us, wherein each of us could resonate with our shared, albeit different, feelings of shame and fear and our strategies of disconnection. It was becoming increasingly "safe to talk" while actually thinking about the other's feelings. I told Maura that I thought her list was "right on the money" and that what remained for us was to look at our series of feelings and reactions in order to better understand what can happen interpersonally in any relationship. She groaned and laughed, asking, "Oh, no! Do we have to? Can't we just move on to something else?"

Over the next several sessions, Maura and I went over this incident in an effort to both reconnect in a deeper, more meaningful way and to understand the complex ebb and flow of feelings and behaviors between two people in a relationship. Maura's experiences growing up and in adulthood did not include bearing relational conflict in the service of mutual growth. As her motto expressed her worldview, the only two options were to conquer or to flee. Our sustained examination of our conflict and the bearing of such emotional uncertainty were new for her and became the substance of a potentially new set of relational images. In a sense, we were engaging together in "making great memories." My consultation with a colleague served some of the same function in the sense of turning a vulnerable acknowledgment of therapeutic uncertainty and reactivity into an opportunity for deepened insight rather than shame. Being able to bring this experience of trust and faith in relationship back to my challenged connection with Maura functioned to open her up to a more authentic and vulnerable representation of her own feelings toward me. This exchange became an empowering cycle of nonshaming mutual empathy that enabled us to safely bring more of ourselves into relationship with one another.

Places of vulnerability are not simply old relational wounds but, rather, old wounds that remain open in the present. In the healthiest sense, people in relationship typically meet in these places of open woundedness in one another and grow from such contact through empathy. In our case, Maura and I met in a place of shared complexity about giving and sacrificing, pieces of which we both brought to the relationship and brought out in one another. While our complicated images were different from one another's, they rendered us similarly confused and vulnerable at times. By bringing into focus these images and their current relational translation between Maura and me, Maura became increasingly able to speak of her relationship with Cara with a greater breadth of feeling. She could acknowledge both her joy at giving her niece a good life as well as the pain this sacrifice has caused her in certain ways. She could look back on the sacrifices she was asked to make in her family around emotional and financial caretaking and address her anger and hurt at the ways in which she has felt unacknowledged and taken for granted. Maura could talk about her desire for help and begin to tackle the associated feelings of shame and weakness that she has carried. She could begin to identify the loneliness she has felt and also perpetuated through her denial of need and adherence to the role of provider as a source of personal empowerment. Maura has perfected the art of hard work and giving, but she has slowly been learning the importance of needing and receiving in a relationship.

THE WIDENING CIRCLE OF EMPATHY

Recently, Maura and her niece had a long conversation about growing up and becoming an adult. Cara told her that she did not want to become an adult, because adults do not seem to have much fun. Rather than challenging this observation, Maura took in its important message and told me about it, realizing her own contribution to that image of adulthood. Maura has always tended to work excessively, has derived most of her "fun" from the challenges and success of business, and can treat life as a series of chores to be tackled and checked off the list. She is beginning to recognize that life needs to be more than work and sacrifice and that she has always been fearful of slowing down and relaxing. This fear is due, in part, to her relational images of poverty and betrayal in the face of relaxed vigilance. Maura wants to change these images for herself and for her relationship with Cara. She wants to let Cara know that she heard her, that she felt Cara's empathic connection, and that that connection has contributed to her growth and the ultimate growth of the relationship with her niece. For Maura, communicating with Cara in this way will be yet another new and perhaps more profound form of giving, one with more meaningful and enduring relational value—a truly "great memory."

REFERENCES

Ehrenberg, D. B. (1974). The intimate edge in therapeutic relatedness. *Contemporary Psychoanalysis, 10*(4), 423–437.

Hartling, L., Rosen, W. B., Walker, M., & Jordan, J. V. (2000). Shame and humiliation: From isolation to relational transformation. *Work in Progress, No. 88.* Wellesley, MA: Stone Center Working Paper Series.

Jordan, J. V. (1985). The meaning of mutuality. *Work in Progress, No. 23.*

Jordan, J. V., Surrey, J. L., & Kaplan, A. G. (1981). Women and empathy: Implications for psychological development and psychotherapy. *Work in Progress, No. 2.* Wellesley, MA: Stone Center Working Paper Series.

Miller, J. B., & Stiver, I. P. (1997). *The healing connection.* Boston: Beacon Press.

Rosen, W. B. (1999). Moments of truth: Notes from a lesbian therapist. *Smith College Studies in Social Work, 69*(2), 293–308.

5

Caring, but Fallible
A Story of Repairing Disconnection

ALICE C. LAWLER

She wrote many poems to me over the course of our work together—some disquieting, some bringing resolution to things we experienced in therapy together. None struck me so much as the one she called "Caring, but Fallible." In it, she spoke about how all the "caretakers" of the past—those who were supposed to "take care" of her—had failed her. The poem came after I, too, had failed her, and she mournfully and eloquently asked that I be a better caretaker, though she was beginning to understand that sometimes I, too, might be caring—but fallible.

I chose "Laura" for this chapter because I believe that our work together illustrates many of the principles of relational–cultural therapy. Sometimes this approach is seen as best used for simple cases, wherein the therapist needs only to listen and be empathic. Laura's situation is complex and challenging. In this chapter I hope to illustrate the many ways the theory and the therapy model on which it is based guided my every step with Laura. It provided a framework and a template for some difficult treatment decisions.

DIAGNOSIS AND BEGINNING CONNECTIONS

Laura came to me about 10 years ago in a state of almost complete psychological disarray. I was acquainted with her because she had, on occasion, asked me to make a presentation on relational–cultural therapy at a conference sponsored by an organization for which she worked.

On the outside, she was bright, articulate, witty, powerful, influential in the community. Inside, she was unraveling emotionally from some extremely difficult life circumstances and from a previous course of therapy that appeared to have been poorly paced, poorly managed, and poorly ended. There was a lot I did not know about Laura when she called me and first asked me to be her therapist. I do not remember struggling a great deal with the decision, perhaps because, like many others, I had only seen Laura at her best—as a competent professional woman.

With Laura's permission, I consulted the previous therapist who had diagnosed Laura with multiple personality disorder (the nomenclature used at that time). Both Laura and the previous therapist recounted stories of cults, murders of babies by Laura's parents and herself, and people in dark robes drinking blood by candlelight. Her previous therapy ended, like many things around this time in her life, dramatically. Laura's rage had become unmanageable both to herself and to her therapist. With some suddenness, the previous therapist let her know that she could no longer work as her therapist, but would give her referrals to other mental health professionals in town if she wanted them. The loss of this relationship was a huge blow to Laura. Unfortunately, its magnitude was matched by the magnitude of the loss of her professional position as well.

Laura was a middle child; she has an older brother and a younger sister who committed suicide when Laura was 21 and the sister was 18. Her sister killed herself at the family home while her parents were out of the country on vacation. Laura's mother suffered from serious and frequent depressions. The most serious occurred after the birth of Laura's younger sister, and it was so severe that she was hospitalized. Her father allegedly physically and sexually abused Laura, but Laura now has some confusion about the veracity of these memories and the extent of the abuse. Laura describes her mother as unpredictable and unavailable—characteristics which hold true to the present. Her father was the gatekeeper—he kept the children away from Mom when she was depressed or drunk and often took her on trips out of the state and out of the country. These frequent trips were a source of intense anxiety for Laura. The multiple disconnections they involved created an intense longing in her for connection and a terrible fear that she was powerless to prevent the disconnections.

Laura first came to see me at the end of back-to-back psychiatric hospitalizations. She was 33 years old and had been married for the previous 6 years. In traditional terms, she might have fit some very pathological diagnoses. But, because practitioners of relational–cultural therapy hesitate to use language that overpathologizes or objectifies the client, I found myself reluctant to use the obvious diagnoses of borderline personality disorder or dissociative identity disorder. Instead, relational–cultural therapy principles led me in a different direction from the beginning. I chose posttraumatic stress disorder, since it seemed clear to me that Laura's destabilization could be traced to several traumatic childhood events, such as the hospitalization of her mother (for postpartum depression) after the birth of her sister when Laura was 3. In making a diagnosis, the relational–cultural therapist looks more carefully at contextual issues and environmental causes of psychopathology, not just at the intrapsychic forces. A cornerstone of the therapy is that the development of psychopathology can be traced to disconnection. This was certainly the case with Laura, and from the beginning, I conceptualized her destabilization as arising from some very serious disconnections early in her life.

Laura was quite knowledgeable about psychological terms, and it proved extremely helpful and calming to her to hear that what was happening to her was posttraumatic stress disorder, rather than the previous diagnoses she had been given, multiple personality disorder and borderline personality disorder. In nonpathologizing language, she could begin to understand some of her intense feelings, overreactions to events, and difficulties trusting others as logical consequences of a series of early traumatic separations.

From the beginning, the therapy veered between periods of profound connection and periods of total disconnection. During the first year, she frequently dissociated during the sessions, sometimes requiring 20–30 minutes of my efforts to bring her back into the room. During these episodes, she would report remembering such things as being made to kill babies, watching others kill babies, or being brutally physically or sexually abused by one of the caretakers from her childhood. These dissociations would take her completely out of connection with me and, I think, also with herself. If we were out of connection, we could not do the reparative work of relational–cultural therapy. In those moments, I would encourage her to look at me, talk to me, stay with me in the room, as she tried to remember the events of the past. This process of helping her stay connected with me and recovering the connection when it was lost is an essential practice of relational–cultural therapy.

As I was able to help her stop the dissociation by slowly and carefully processing the content of some of the images and emphasizing the importance of her remembering without reexperiencing, a new symptom emerged—somaticization. As the dissociation decreased, the conversion of her psychological pain into bodily symptoms increased. In the fall of our first year together, she began to feel numbness in her arms and legs, then an increasing inability to walk, which she later came to believe was multiple sclerosis. She had persistent eye problems, which she feared would become blindness; she also had neck pain, shoulder pain, and headaches. Her medicine cabinet bulged as she found physicians to prescribe various medications (many of them, powerful narcotics and pain-killers).

THE FIRST DISCONNECTION AND REPAIR

One of the primary dynamics of relational–cultural therapy is the fundamental relational flow of movement from connection to disconnection to reconnection. Laura and I played out this movement many times during our work together. We had literally dozens of disconnections—it was impossible not to fail her, given the magnitude of her need. The first major disconnection occurred around 10 months into the therapy. As I mentioned before, I had often been asked to make presentations on relational–cultural therapy at the conference sponsored by her now-former employer. Since leaving the job, she had developed a very negative attitude toward the employer. Around the time of my beginning to see Laura, I had, without much careful thought, agreed to present a program at the following year's conference.

I had some initial suspicion that Laura would not be very happy about my participation. But as the months wore on, she spent much of our therapy time raging at her former coworkers. I began to squirm more and more in my chair about the fact that I had agreed to participate again in their conference. It was one thing to hear her rage at her previous staff and her previous therapist, but I dreaded being the object of her rage. I had written at the top of my notes for four or five sessions, "Remember to tell her about the presentation" and then "forgotten," or "felt that there wasn't time," or that the crisis of the day took too much of our energy and she was not ready to hear this news. I made excuses for not telling her this critical piece of information. I felt more and more out of connection with her. We could not be in real relationship as long as I avoided speaking the truth to her. And until we were in real relationship, the therapy would be stalled.

One of my own relational images is that others' rage and anger toward me can be devastating and overwhelming. My own fears got in the way of my handling this revelation better. I think I could have avoided some of the distress I caused her if I had not been so afraid myself and had spoken up sooner.

Finally, when I could wait no longer, I told her. I explained that I had made a commitment and it was not one on which I felt I could reneg. She was shocked, appalled, enraged, disbelieving that I would do such a thing. How could I betray her? I was indeed just like all the rest of them—the caretakers who had failed her, especially her mother and her previous therapist. I, too, could not be trusted or believed. I, too, caused the inevitable "whiplash," a word she used to describe what it frequently felt like when her mother would be sometimes caring and later rejecting, withholding, or unavailable. This event almost ended our work together and, truly, by this time, there was a part of me that would have been relieved to see it end.

Laura was retraumatized, a feeling she would experience over and over during our work together. She became flooded again with memories and flashbacks; she again frequently dissociated in our sessions and outside of them, and frequently somaticized her psychological issues. In this period, she had a long series of accidents and illnesses and traveled from emergency room to emergency room.

RELATIONAL IMAGES

Let us look more closely at the moment of disconnection between Laura and me and consider the underlying relational images. Relational images are notions we form, beginning in childhood, about how the world operates. They are often based on limited or distorted information or on information that is seen only through the child's eyes. I believe that one of Laura's relational images was that her needs could never be met adequately—that if she placed her trust in someone, like Mom or Dad, she would be betrayed. People may pretend that they care or they may care inconsistently, but, ultimately, they will not be there for her. Laura used to get sick or injured in sports activities when she was a child, usually around the time that her mother and father were about to leave for a big trip out of town. She was testing them—would they forego the trip to help her recuperate? Would they go anyway, leaving her to get well on her own? Usually, at least from her perspective, it was the latter. Then they would come home bearing "guilt" gifts—and she would refuse to accept them.

In later life, with this issue unresolved, it became impossible for anyone to adequately meet her needs. Always, at some point, there would be that whiplash, that disappointment, that sense of betrayal, that disconnection that would evoke Laura's rage. At every turn, she felt retraumatized. When her previous therapist suddenly tried to put some limits on a therapy gone out of control, Laura felt disconnected and enraged. When I, whom she had come to trust, told her of my agreement to give a presentation for the conference, she felt betrayed, enraged, and disconnected. Mom, the previous therapist, and I all merged together in Laura's mind. Her reactions to even small disappointments in the present were experienced as overwhelming, and she felt very little ability to modulate her emotions.

She would often say that things were all blending together, that she could not separate the abuse of the past from the pain of the present. Our work consisted of my repeatedly trying to help her separate me from Mom and from the previous therapist. Helping her to stay in the room with me, to be present in our real-time relationship, was a large part of our work together. If she could separate us one from the other, she could then have a better chance of managing her reaction to the present event. Together we could try to untangle the knot of reality and memory that had been tied so tightly in the previous work. I refer to a "knot" because the poorly paced work on Laura's memories and the powerful dynamics it evoked had blurred the line, perhaps irrevocably, between what really had happened to her and her psychological construct of the events of her childhood. The two had truly become tied in a knot.

At the heart of Laura's work was and, in many ways, still is, her relationship with her mother. She expressed her personal paradox at the end of our first year of work: "I want to be held by my mother, and I want to throw her down the stairs." How could I metaphorically hold Laura—because she so desperately wanted and needed to be held by a solid and consistent mother—and at the same time not create the dangerous dependency and expectation, which, when failed, would trigger her rageful desire to throw me down my rather high and steep stairs?

As in the previous therapy, Laura experienced a powerful maternal transference with me. The two women before me had failed her. How could I not fall into the same trap? How could I establish a healthy, caring connection with Laura that also allowed for me to be fallible—to make mistakes, to miss the mark, to say something that fell outside of the very narrow range of responses she required of me? That was my challenge for the first 5 years of our work together. The task was to change the flawed relational image she had formed through reparative experience of the therapeutic relationship. Yes, she might be betrayed by those in whom she placed her trust, but equally likely is that those caretakers simply made mistakes, or were insensitive, or misread a situation—and in reality, they *did* care about her.

After things had calmed down between us, she brought me a poem she had written in which she talked about wanting someone "caring, but fallible." I think that this expression marked her first step in her being able to see events from another person's perspective. It was her first step in her being able to reconnect with me, something that she desperately wanted to do. "Caring, but fallible" became almost a mantra for us over the years, although she never really liked my going back to those words, and she would roll her eyes whenever I did so. Nevertheless, she always knew that caring, but fallible was the best she could hope for, and if she could accept it, then she would, quite literally, survive.

I asked her during one of our therapy sessions to trust me, to trust that I could help her in spite of my failings. She wrote the poem "your request" in response:

your request

it sounds simple.
just two words,
with three more implied:
"trust me"
"let me in."

why?
because the name of the game
has changed.
it's no longer
What's That Memory.
it's now
Life or Death.

the tune was changed,
the tone was changed.
someone, somewhere
upped the ante.

"trust me;
let me in."
if i keep you out?
could be i die.

are you that important:
am i?
you must think you're important
if letting you in, if trusting you
is the key to my life right now.
or you must think i'm important.
or that our connection is.

ah! that's the right answer.
the "connection."
a tainted theory right now
for the author.

but also a dilemma.
the author doesn't want only
posthumous recognition
of her life.

and that's the current script
in her hands,
without connection.

so . . . trust you.
let you in.
quite a request.

i, too, have a request.
help me dismantle
the minefield.

letting someone in
is not that easy.

but then,
i think you know that.
you found the minefield.

BOUNDARIES

At this point in our work, relational–cultural therapy guided several key treatment decisions. One of them concerned an explicit discussion of boundaries. The word is redefined in relational–cultural therapy to mean places of connection rather than places of separation. I always tried to hold firmly the "boundaries" of our time together, as well as to remind her of why those clear boundaries were so important to us and to our relationship. In her home, growing up, the rules were chaotic, unpredictable, constantly changing, confusing, and disorienting. In her previous therapy, sessions could go on for many minutes, and sometimes hours, past their scheduled stopping point. In our therapy, I told her, I would define the rules as clearly as I could and explain explicitly why it is important that we both respect those rules. This explanation included more explicit discussions of the ways in which her boundaries were violated in the past, pointing out the inconsistencies in the caretaking she had received and the confusion she must feel as a result, being clear that our context in therapy would be different—the rules would be clearer, the process more consistent, and the seemingly unmanageable feelings more contained.

Instead of seeing boundaries as points of separation and confrontation, we came to talk about them as places of connection—places where we could meet and figure out together what would be psychologically healthy for her. We tended our boundaries with a sense of mutuality—not from the stance that I, as the therapist, had power over her, but that we shared the power inherent in our relationship and could together make decisions together about what was in her best interest.

AUTHENTICITY

Another decision I made was to be as honest and authentic with her as possible, tell her about my own decision-making process when I thought that information would be helpful to her. At some point after we had discussed boundaries, I asked her to write about what she thought was the turning point for her in what I said. She wrote:

> It seemed to take for *fucking* ever, but at some point, you said that if you had to do it over again, you might make a different decision about doing the workshop. . . . What those words said to me was that something about my feelings/needs touched you—again, a new experience for me. The beginning seed of the caring-but-fallible concept.

She said that she felt cared about, but was not sure that she could trust the caring. When I had identified myself as fallible, could she trust the caring? That I might have considered making a different decision made an enormous impact on her. My acknowledgment of that possibility helped her see that she did, indeed, have an impact on me. It is almost as though my fallibility became a precondition for trust. My fallibility also allowed us both to experience the mutuality of our relationship. In this exchange, we played out that powerful relational–cultural therapy principle that if a client feels that he or she has affected the therapist in some way, then he or she can *move* in the therapy.

THE SECOND DISCONNECTION AND REPAIR

The second and third years of therapy were fraught with difficulties; as the dissociation abated, the physical symptoms became central—continuing eye problems, fears about MS (she began using a wheelchair), accidents, then a seizure disorder. She also experienced frequent suicidal episodes. In addition to the usual safety and containment procedures, I tried to help her understand the triggers for these episodes. Slowly, I tried to help her begin to look at the possibility that some of these physiological symptoms might be manifestations of her psychological distress.

She hated these sessions—there was a narrow band of acceptable responses she could tolerate from me. I tried to be as supportive and empathic as possible, and, at the same time, to stand still, to serve as a kind of anchor for her as she felt her own life spinning out of control. Particularly with a client such as Laura, the relational practice of standing still, of providing solid, mindful attention, is an important one.

Her longtime physician, whom I'll call Carl, and I were each closing in on the psychosomatic angle and the possibility that Laura was experiencing some form of conversion reaction. This focus made Laura nervous and edgy with me. The issue of being believed was a big one for her—since Mom and Dad had never believed that she was really sick unless they could see a broken bone on the X-ray. (She once obliged by breaking her knee in a high school sports event moments before they were to leave town.) Yet I felt that I would be doing her a disservice if I did not raise these possibilities.

We were in one of these periods of tension, and she had grown more and more suicidal. Her husband, who had grown weary of these suicidal episodes, brought her to a session one morning. She had begun to have people accompany her because by now she was in a wheelchair. The session was a difficult one. I spent half the time trying to figure out if she needed to be hospitalized for her safety and half the time trying to nudge her into seeing some of what was going on in her body as connected to what was going on in her mind.

As she was leaving, Laura asked me to promise not to tell her husband that she was suicidal. I reluctantly promised—partly because she had so earnestly asked me to, partly because I knew her husband was weary of these suicidal phases, and perhaps mostly because it was the end of the session and I wanted to avoid a big conflict with her over this issue. I then walked out into the waiting room with her as she wheeled herself out there. When my eyes met the husband's eyes, I said, almost involuntarily, "You should be careful and watch out for Laura's safety." I was a bit stunned myself that these words had come out of my mouth. In the moment of promising her that I would not tell her husband about her suicidality, I had truly meant it. But in the waiting room, with her about to leave for several days, I felt this huge responsibility to tell him so that he could be watchful of her. Although I had tried to say it obliquely, all three of us knew instantly that my words meant she was suicidal. Laura screamed at me: "I can't believe you just said that! You have violated my confidentiality."

As well as one can storm out to a car in a wheelchair, Laura did so. Somewhat dangerously, she got herself and her wheelchair down the stairs and around the house and into her car. I followed, in some disbelief myself that I had said what I said. She raged at me in the parking lot, while I tried to both calm her down and explain as best I could why I had said what I said. I explained her choices: She could agree to be hospitalized for her suicidality, or she could agree to see me the next day. I encouraged her husband to call emergency services if he could not calm Laura. She agreed to come for a session the next day. Her husband followed silently and dejectedly, exhausted from years of this chaotic pattern of behavior.

Laura left several phone messages that night, threatening to make a complaint to my licensing board for violating her confidentiality, saying she wanted three closure sessions and the final bill, talking about funeral plans and her despair. On one message, she said, "You've made it clear that you've reached your limits. So if you don't want to listen to this anymore, hang up. I don't give a rip. It was not okay what you did, and I'm sure you'll decide that this is all me. You won't take any responsibility for this."

Rereading my notes from the couple of months following that disconnection was like a PTSD response for me. Laura punished and punished and punished me for my betrayals, for my suggestion of psychosomatic possibilities and my words to her husband in the waiting room. She could not stop talking about it, yet she constantly resented having to use her therapy time to do so. I remember feeling psychologically abused by her during this period, dreading our appointments and phone calls. I tried to walk that tricky line between acknowledging the validity of her feelings and holding to my understanding of why I had done what I had done.

In the midst of it all, she attacked my relational and feminist allegiances. She said that I pathologized her, that I had all the power, that I did not practice mutuality, that I was not a safe person, that I used my power in a damaging way by bringing up the possibility of a conversion reaction. She berated me for being inconsistent—that I first said she was courageous in dealing with these things and that now I said she was avoiding them. Every effort to talk about what had transpired between us on that fateful day was seen as analyzing and pathologizing and keeping her from talking about what was really important to her. We could not go forward, I thought, until we got some resolution of that event, and she could not get any resolution of it until I was willing to leave it behind and attend to her needs in the present. Then she talked about how this therapy felt one-sided, and the personal risk was all on her side—that I used a lot of "white male therapist in disguise" statements and that she would like to be with a feminist therapist. She had thought that I was one, but it was now clear that I was not.

She came in one day saying that she had read a book about therapeutic impasse in therapy, reviewed by Irene Stiver, in which it said that the client's perception is important. She felt that we were at a therapeutic impasse and that she did not have a therapist—that she could not come to me for support, that we had a place of battle here. She came into my office as though she were wearing armor. I could not make any connection with her. I tried to be empathic, to do what relational–cultural therapy calls "honoring her strategies of disconnection." These are the ways in which our clients try to protect themselves—sort of like "defense mechanisms" in traditional language, but they are ways our clients try and keep people at a distance in order to keep themselves safe. This was no easy task at this point! I tried to help her understand the dynamics of what had transpired between us: the repetition of the betrayal and the intensity of the feeling, because it brought back all of the previous betrayals.

She also brought in two of the Stone Center Working Papers, "A Relational Reframing of Therapy" (Miller & Stiver, 1991) and "Courage in Connection: Conflict, Compassion, and Creativity" (Jordan, 1990). She had reread them in the light of our disconnection and written in red all over them how consistently and wholeheartedly I had failed to live up to the standards of relational–cultural practice.

For months at a time, I questioned myself. Was she right on some level? Had I been nonrelational in my treatment of her? Had my anger and frustration with her come out in nontherapeutic and pathologizing ways? Had I retraumatized her? At times during this period, I felt very discouraged—certain that other psychologists in my community would do a much better job with Laura, that I had made a series of mistakes and missteps that may have made it impossible for our therapeutic work to continue. I felt, at times, foolish, defeated, a failure—and I relied heavily on a couple of colleagues to keep my own energy alive for the continued work with her.

Several things helped us reconnect. First, I did not get sucked into the maelstrom with her. Second, and perhaps most importantly, I owned my part of that terrible interaction. I, of course, could not deny that I had said what I said, but I tried to help her understand that it came from a caring place. I was worried about her—caring, but fallible—the old mantra again. I tried not to pathologize her or blame her or see the terrible outcome of that session as all her fault. My comments regarding the somaticizing also came from caring, because I was beginning to see some of her medical emergencies as dangerous and self-destructive.

Third, I empathized with her distress and tried to honor her powerful strategies of disconnection. I tried to get in her shoes and feel how frightened she must be, how unsafe she must feel, that she felt that the only safe thing to do was to push people away with her rage.

RELATIONAL PARADOX

Here again, relational–cultural therapy guided my work. I knew that she was living the relational paradox: that in her deep desire for connection, she often kept large parts of herself out of connection and engaged in powerful strategies of disconnection. So I tried to empathize with both sides of the paradox—the part that so deeply and desperately wanted to connect, especially with important women in her life (her mother, her previous therapist, me), and the other side that was scared and terrified of that connection as dangerous, consuming, intolerable to lose. We talked about her fear that her rage would destroy others, consume them, and how she would then sometimes turn that rage toward herself—resulting in these long periods of suicidality.

Fourth, I challenged her attempt to sabotage the whole therapeutic endeavor because of this one situation, pointing out that she was throwing out years of good, important, solid work as though they never existed and as though we had no previously connected relationship. This practice of complete disconnection, so prevalent in her family, was one that we had to watch out for continually, both in the therapy relationship and in her relationships with others.

Slowly, over many months, the tenor of the sessions changed; she would arrive in a slightly softer state. She decided that I had made a mistake, and that she would wait and see if I would continue to make a series of mistakes before she quit therapy with me. Finally, in one session, she was able to cry with me again—about her fears that this therapy was going the same way as the previous therapy (some of my explanations were similar to those given by the previous therapist). She felt scared and sad: "I don't know how to make this work again. I need to talk about things. I have a life, and I need your help."

THE THIRD DISCONNECTION AND REPAIR

Laura and I had one last serious disconnection. Laura's physical symptoms continued to worsen. In the fifth year of the therapy, Carl, her long-time physician and friend (and supplier of all kinds of medications, narcotic and otherwise) suddenly, and without acknowledgment to anyone, retired from medicine. This devastating loss sent her into another long period of suicidal depression. Here is a poem, which she called "Buoys," that she wrote about Carl and me during this period:

> First the endless undertow;
> drowning, drowning—only
> coming up for air enough
> to keep me alive . . .
> and to connect with one
> soothing blue buoy
> bobbing in the churning
> waters—there to connect
> with, hang on to, until

the undertow ruled again.
Finally, in my view,
came a second similar
buoy.

The power of both, generally
always there
led to more freedom
than I'd ever had.

Using the strength offered
by both, I came to shore.
And they came to shore,
and alive as people—
who meant well, who
cared, who taught . . .
always patiently.
Caring, but fallible—
yet infallible enough for
me to integrate me through
them. . . .

And then
one day,
one of the buoys found
himself in an undertow.

And was swept out to
sea.
Vanished. Gone.
All his wisdom shared with
me about self-care,
revealed
Like the Wizard of Oz,
A great and mighty voice—
who was found to be blustering,
and tosseled. . . .

And so,
the writer,
She looks at the other buoy
come to life.
She knows only too well
that history repeats itself. . . .
Why go back to the
interpreter of the psyche?
Why not just GO.

A colleague of Carl's informed her that Carl's records indicated that everything for which he treated her was psychologically based, and this colleague refused to give her any further narcotic-type medication. This loss, along with my departure for an annual conference trip, plus the news that her parents were leaving the country for a vacation, set the stage for the psychological drama she then enacted. She came into a session saying that she had ovarian cancer. I had become more and more convinced that she had no legitimate physiological condition. As her "condition" worsened, I leaned harder and harder on her to allow me to speak to her oncologist. She continually refused. She stopped coming to sessions because of her health and because she hated my asking permission to talk with her doctors. For much of this time period, we had weekly telephone sessions.

When I look back on this period of our work, I think that what most challenged me was how to stay in authentic connection with Laura. Relational–cultural therapy requires authenticity, but as I grew more and more skeptical of her physical symptoms, she grew more and more afraid. As she got more frightened, her tolerance for my responses narrowed to the point where I felt that the only way to keep the relationship alive was for me to be inauthentic and "believe" that she was terminally ill. Paradoxically, I felt that the only way to keep the connection with her was to be really out of connection with her. It was a predicament that tormented me for several months.

During this time, I also started reading everything I could get my hands on about psychosomatic illness. I found myself in the dilemma posed by Steven Dubovsky (1997) in his book *Mind–Body Deceptions: The Psychosomatics of Everyday Life*: "The answer to this question—'Is the patient *really* ill?'—is never clear when dealing with somatization, because the fantasy of what is in the body can never be entirely separated from the truth of what is in the mind" (p. 100).

The final debacle finally occurred. She felt that she was dying and had gathered friends and some family around her. Someone called the doctor's office to inquire about hospice care and found that there was no record of her ever having been there. I had suspected this for a long time, but her clients and friends had truly believed that she was dying. She became enraged that they had called the doctor. She got suicidal and both her friends and I called emergency services to get her committed. When police arrived, she collected herself enough to convince them that she was not suicidal.

When the crisis subsided, Laura returned to therapy and we began the long and continuing process of trying to figure out what happened to cause this drama to unfold in the self-destructive way in which it did. She asked me to help her through the minefield she had created and to help her not lose her mind in the process. Her closest friends, some of whom she had been friends with for many years, severed their relationships with her. This was another devastating loss for her. She feared losing me, but, again, with the guidance of relational–cultural therapy, we were able to sit together and figure out how to repair the relationship between us.

CONCLUSION

For the first 5 years of my work with Laura, I sought consultation from someone who worked within a much more traditional psychodynamic model of psychotherapy. Though his approach was different from mine, he provided a valuable and useful counterpoint. Although we may have used different language and different conceptualizations, our conversations were extremely useful to me. He helped me do what I needed to do. In his language, it was "setting limits"; in the language of relational–cultural therapy, it was explaining to Laura the need to contain our sessions, to meet her at the boundary and decide together what would be best for her and why. One of my office partners also provided the voice of reason and equanimity. He anchored me when Laura tried to send us both out into the storms of her emotional life. I could not have done this work alone. I could not have stayed in relationship with Laura without the help of these important supporting relationships.

A second point is that I never stopped liking Laura. As is obvious from some of her words that I have quoted here, she is an immensely talented and gifted woman.

Thirdly, I think that Laura and I have lived out the essence of relational–cultural theory. We have gone from connection, to disconnection, to reconnection again, and we have done so in major ways (as explained above) and in minor ways countless times. During the many years of our work together, we have done this dance over and over. Ever so slowly, but surely, she has been able to experience a healthy relationship with me. And, more importantly, she has been able to take what she has learned here and transfer it to that relationship that is still the most important one of her life—with her mother.

I want to close with Laura' s words in this regard. She continues to struggle to figure out how to have a healthy relationship with her mother, who continues to struggle to figure out how to have a healthy relationship with her daughter. Her mother continues to come and go—inconsistently, imperfectly, unpredictably—a pattern so painful and so familiar to Laura. Interestingly, there is a kind of parallel in her words: Just as I so often stood still in my interactions with her, she feels the need to be the anchor, to be the still one, in the relationship with her mother. I will close with her words in this poem:

easy come, easy go

you come into my life
    when you want,

you leave my life
    when you want

and the rhythm knows only
    your whim.

tolerated, sometimes, in a friend.
expected, sometimes, in a child.
unacceptable in a mother.

and yet,
    what is there
    for me to do?

there is only
    standing still
while you whirl.

i'm still standing,
    still.

and now,
    that is good enough
    for me.

REFERENCES

Dubovsky, S. L. (1997). *Mind–body deceptions: The psychosomatics of everyday life.* New York: Norton.

Jordan, J. V. (1990). Courage in connection: Conflict, compassion, and creativity. *Work in Progress, No. 45.* Wellesley, MA: Stone Center Working Paper Series.

Miller, J. B., & Stiver, I. P. (1991). A relational reframing of therapy. *Work in Progress, No. 52.* Wellesley, MA: Stone Center Working Paper Series.

6

Reflections on Life, Loss, and Resilience

DANA L. COMSTOCK

Carin was referred to me by her obstetrician after the death of her 3-month-old infant son "Noah." I knew her doctor quite well. I have a small private practice, in addition to working as a counselor educator, and have seen many of his patients to deal with obstetrical complications and infant loss. In fact, I had been his patient and had developed this specialty by default, not by choice. The themes woven throughout this case stem from the convergence of my life circumstances with Carin's. It is about the challenges we faced trying to connect through impenetrable grief, our mutual strategies for survival, and our growth and resilience.

For Carin, Noah's death was devastating, untimely, unjust, and so much more. She and her family had already suffered the loss of her first baby, a daughter, "Meg," who was stillborn at full term. After Meg, Carin had a son, Benjamin, who was 2 years old when we began our work. Noah, her third child, began having problems shortly after birth. Before his death he had suffered through several surgeries to correct bowel obstructions and was suffering from other neurological problems that caused him to have frequent seizures.

During his short life his seizures became progressively worse, turning into infantile spasms, as many as 20 a day. To treat the seizures, he was initially given prednisone, which did not work. Interestingly, he was given his first dose of an experimental drug, which did seem to work, the same day he died. Noah had survived one previous stop breathing episode (SBE) and, at the time of his death, was being fed through a stomach tube. While Ariel, Carin's husband, worked and coordinated Benjamin's care, Carin spent countless hours with Noah during his hospital stays.

One of the most difficult aspects of caring for Noah was the absence of a specific diagnosis, the fact of no guarantees, and no hint as to the quality of his life for the moment or into the near or distant future. The stress became unbearable. Overwhelmed and exhausted, Carin took the advice of a friend and reluctantly made an appointment to see a psychiatrist for help. The psychiatrist, whom I will call Dr. Thompson, prescribed a low dose of Prozac and recommended that Carin also seek counseling. Because Carin was simply exhausted and overwhelmed by the idea of seeing yet another mental health provider, she asked Dr. Thompson if she would see her for counseling. This was not customary for Dr. Thompson's type of practice, but she reluctantly agreed.

A LIVING NIGHTMARE

The week prior to Carin's first scheduled visit for counseling with Dr. Thompson was filled with more of the continual demands required for Noah's care. Still trying to care for her 2-year-old son, Carin worked out a sleeping arrangement that would accommodate the needs of both Benjamin and Noah. Carin decided that instead of co-sleeping with Noah, she would co-sleep with Benjamin while Noah slept next to the bed in a small bassinet. Ariel slept in another room to avoid the frequent awakenings, because he was working full time during this period. The sleeping arrangements worked wonderfully the first night.

In the morning, however, Carin noticed that Noah had a red raw spot on the tip of his nose where he had apparently rubbed against the mesh lining of the bassinet during a seizure in the night. To prevent him from rubbing his nose raw again the second night, she placed a thin, softer blanket over the mesh lining and tucked the ends under the mattress.

After going to sleep the second night, Carin was awakened around 1:00 A.M. by the alarm sounding from Noah's apnea monitor. Horrified, and knowing he needed to be resuscitated, she screamed for Ariel. Ariel began to work to get Noah breathing again while she called 911. She paced back and forth in her nightgown on their balcony, desperately searching the parking lot for the ambulance. At some point she made it to her bathroom to change her clothes, all the while pleading with the person on the other end of the phone to please tell the ambulance to hurry!

She sat in silence in the front of the ambulance on the way to the hospital. She knew enough about the coded language being communicated to the hospital that things were not going well. Once in the ER, she waited anxiously as they continued working on Noah. Ariel finally arrived with his mother. Shortly thereafter, a nurse came to tell them that although they had done all they could, Noah had died, probably due to a compilation of catastrophic factors related to his seizure disorder. In the face of shock and disbelief, they were given Noah's lifeless body. Carin recalls apologizing to Ariel's mother. She also remembers noticing a red, raw spot on his nose, which elicited a comment from her mother-in-law. Carin had not noticed it during the emergency, and no one on the hospital staff had remarked about it. She described feeling deeply ashamed of this "mark."

Carin and Ariel were left with Noah's body while the coroner's office was called. The police were also called, as is customary in cases of infant death. Carin could overhear the hospital staff telling the officer how her son had been very ill. The officer asked very few questions, offered his condolences, and left. It took hours for the coroner to arrive. It took so long that the hospital staff offered to take Noah's body from Carin, as it had started to become cold and stiff. Although this bothered her, she chose to keep him with her anyway.

She was aware that the ER staff had discretely worked to hide this scene from other ER patients by ushering them to a room off the main hallway, where they were able to close the curtains and obstruct the view into the room. It was not for their privacy, really, as they had been as comfortable as possible, under the circumstances, where they were. Life was moving on, and they needed to get out of the way. The coroner did make it, finally. Noah's body was covered and taken away. Carin was assured this was not the last time she would see him. It was morning by now, the day of her first scheduled therapy appointment with Dr. Thompson.

Carin shares what happened next.

> "I called the woman shrink I had met only once before, on the day we had agreed to meet again. Her father's cheerful voice answered the phone, and I asked to speak to her. After a short hold, she came on the line. Her voice was icy and angry. You see, I was calling her at the time we had agreed to meet, and she was not happy with me. She quickly changed her tone of voice when I told her why I had not met with her at our arranged time. 'Noah died last night,' I heard myself whisper in a hoarse voice. This conversation is cloudy to me, but I do recall it being a lengthy one.
>
> "I remember apologizing to her for keeping her on the phone. She asked if I had begun the medication. When I replied 'No,' she again became impatient with me. I told her I hadn't even picked it up from the pharmacy, because I was afraid I would take the whole bottle. She implored me to begin taking it and again asked me to

call her if I had any thoughts of harming myself. She even gave me her home number, which I wrote on my hand in ink.

"We got back to our apartment late that night. Right away I saw the bassinet standing prominently on the bed. It had been cast aside by the paramedics in a mad rush to work on Noah. I felt it was mocking me, and I was drawn to it right away.

"Ariel and my mother were busy with Benjamin, so I slowly crept closer and closer to the bed. I was afraid to go near it, afraid not to go near it. I moved it cautiously down from its resting place on our bed and anxiously peered into the cradle. My heart was pounding so hard I was afraid Ariel would hear it and come in. Gathering all the courage I could, I reached in and took the soft blue blanket from the bed and saw immediately what I had feared all morning. There it was, a small, bloodied trail that ended in what appeared to be a milk explosion. My breath drew in, I felt sick, and I pulled the blanket to my heart. My God, what had I done?

"I quickly got into bed, clothes and all, clutching the incriminating blanket like a criminal with her murder weapon, until the house was quiet. While Ariel slept, I wondered how I was going to explain to him that I had killed Noah—that he had suffocated, seized face first into the blanket I had put there to protect him. How? The only answer I kept coming back to was to get out of the house with the evidence.

"Around 4:00 in the morning, I was confident I could make my escape, and I quietly crept out of bed with my shameful piece of fabric. I tiptoed into the kitchen, touching the countertop until I struck my car keys. My mother lay feet from me, asleep on the sofa. I slipped out the door and quickly made my way to my waiting car. Having made a quick getaway, I began driving. I didn't know what to do or where to go. I clutched the blanket, that sad reminder of what I had done, tighter and tighter. I didn't cry. I didn't yell. I was on a mission. Finally, as I was driving slowly down San Pedro Avenue, an all-night Walgreen's beckoned to me. 'Come in,' it seemed to say to me. I listened. As I left with my purchase, the clerk said rather cheerfully, 'Have a nice day.'"

In this whole mess of events, Carin remembers just wanting "to sleep." She returned to her mother-in-law's home early that morning. Surrounded by family, she made her way to a quiet spot in the house. Before lying down, she took a number of Tylenol and washed them down with vodka. Her family discovered her several hours later and she was admitted into the hospital for attempted suicide under the care of her obstetrician.

"After a brief but humiliating stay in the hospital, I was released to attend Noah's funeral. I had succeeded in missing the visitation and prayer service, but not the actual funeral. Looking back, I think I not only did not want to tell Ariel about the blanket, but I also did not want to attend another funeral like the one I had sadly been forced to attend just 5 short years ago for Meg, our stillborn daughter.

"Following the funeral, which to this day remains an emotionless vacuum of time, all I wanted to do was sleep. Ariel was reticent to let me, but I reassured him I would be fine, and he left me alone. I drifted into a deep sleep, until all of a sudden I was awakened by a gentle prod.

"Ariel told me the police were downstairs ready to escort me back to the hospital. Apparently my family had agreed to take me back to the hospital following the funeral, and when I did not return, the hospital staff reported me to the police. They informed them that I was a threat to myself. I was incredulous and did not want to go. Finally, after much discussion, I went with them and checked back into the hospital. I felt like a complete freak.

"Obtaining approval from the hospital for my final discharge was quite difficult. In an effort to make plans for follow-up care, my father contacted the psychiatrist. To my horror, she refused to see me again. She felt I had been 'noncompliant' and flat out refused to continue working with me. Being told I was no longer Dr. Thompson's patient, a doctor I had seen only once, made me feel embarrassed, ashamed, angry, and guilty.

"I was embarrassed because I felt I had been unfairly labeled. I was ashamed because I had done something stupid and reckless. I was angry because I suspected my relationships with my caregivers had been sabotaged, and I felt guilty for being away from Benjamin so long and for risking 'being away' from him permanently.

"I had put a lot of trust in Dr. Thompson, trust that I don't give away easily. I felt very betrayed by that trust when she wasn't able, or willing, to give me the benefit of a doubt. Perhaps she was afraid I would really and truly succeed in killing myself, and she would be held liable. But if that's the case, how can any physician ever treat any patient? It seems to me that, out of fear, the entire medical profession could shut down, and then the fear of lawsuits could really kill someone!"

Carin quickly learned that the mental health profession does not tolerate noncompliant, suicidal patients. She had breeched an agreement and was now labeled untrustworthy, manipulative, and attention seeking, and was certainly thought of as suspicious, maybe even "borderline."

Whether or not Dr. Thompson's decision was self-protective, it damaged Carin in a way that we are still working to repair.

SECOND CHANCES

It was Ariel who made the call, which I was expecting, because I had already been briefed by Carin's referring obstetrician. Carin and Ariel, both in their early 30s, came in together for the first visit. It was difficult for them to rehash the details of their trauma yet again. What Carin remembers most about our first session was feeling put at ease by my telling her that I was the mother of a 1-year old and that I, too, had lost a baby. I shared this information because I wanted her to know we would be skipping the part where I ask, "What is it like to lose a baby?" We would use our energy in other areas. There is a regrettable knowing between those who have lost children, an underground experience shared only by those who have "been there." Carin describes it as something "special."

The focus of that first session was Carin's sense of responsibility for Noah's death and Ariel's concern that she might try to kill herself again. Because of this concern, I began doing individual work with Carin. Consistent with relational–cultural theory, my first goal was to help her develop *self-empathy*. She had negated everything she had done for Noah as a mother who had barely had time to recover from childbirth. In short, she blamed herself for Noah's death and was completely out of touch with the countless self-sacrifices she had made.

During our first meeting, I recall having felt very confident about my abilities to help Carin and Ariel. I felt I knew some of what her experience was like as a young mother struggling with the loss of a baby. Fueling my sense of confidence was the experience of my own loss. It had been over 2 years since I had experienced sudden and unexpected pregnancy complications. In my case, complications ensued after I discovered that my cervix had dilated painlessly and prematurely—a typical pattern for those with a diagnosis of "incompetent cervix." After every attempt was made to reverse the cervical dilation, I developed an infection, went into labor, and found myself holding the lifeless body of my daughter, Samantha, who was born still and very premature. Like Carin, I too had blamed myself, and my body, for Samantha's death.[1]

Several weeks after the loss of Samantha, my pain came to a peak in a fleeting episode of psychotic grief, which, for me, gave new meaning to

---

[1]Dana Comstock writes about her loss in "The Initiation." In J. A. Kottler (Ed.), *Counselors finding their way* (2002, pp. 31–34). Alexandria, VA: American Counseling Association.

the saying "I think I'm going crazy." It was at that point that, like Carin, I sought psychiatric help and counseling. Personally, I felt a lot of shame for needing help at all; somewhere along the way I uncovered an image I held of myself as someone who was supposed to know how to handle whatever came her way, no matter the context. I am certain that my training as a mental health provider had something to do with my having developed this image, as it had worked its way into my personal and professional life. Looking back, this image seems so obviously naïve yet dangerously common, readily acceptable, and very easy to slip back into.

To make a long story short, much of my grief work centered around my learning to accept my vulnerabilities, which, in turn, allowed me to dismantle much of my shame around needing help. As a result, I became more comfortable with who I was, both personally and professionally. I also believed that I was better able to simply accept others for who they were and their pain in whatever shape it needed to take. Given the depths of my own growth, I could not imagine how I could have been any more prepared to connect with Carin around her loss. Once again, I felt I was ready to handle whatever came my way.

OUR JOURNEY BEGINS

Having a "sense of preparedness" would seem to be a good thing. Yet looking back, I am aware of how my confidence impeded my ability to clearly think through the goals I began to set for Carin. To be as clear as possible about how we started off, I only looked at what challenges might arise for Carin in our therapeutic relationship. I did not give much thought to my own challenges or to those of our relationship. Relational–cultural theory is very clear about the dangers of one-way thinking. As someone who considers herself a practitioner of relational–cultural therapy, I confess this early mistake with some shame and frustration. Initially, I was confident I was asking all the right questions: What challenges will Carin face in therapy? Who is she in this relationship and what will she become? How will she grow and change?

Because I felt so confident, I failed to engage in more relational two-way thinking and neglected to ask myself the similar round of questions: What will be *my* challenges in this relationship? Who am I and what will I become through this experience? How will I grow and change? With regard to our relationship I could have asked: How will our shared experiences shape our relational dynamics and impact our development of relational resilience and mutual growth? In all fairness, I could not have expected myself to answer any of these questions, but looking back, having merely *asked* them would have better prepared me to take in the answers as they emerged. Given that relationships are never static, we hit the ground running, and our journey began.

It was not long before Carin, in the midst of her grief, started to talk about having another baby. I was tentative about, even frightened by, the idea, and her obstetrician shared my concern. It was now 5 months since Noah's birth and barely 2 months since his death. As it turned out, Carin conceived right away, and with her new pregnancy came a whole new set of concerns. In the first month of her pregnancy, Ariel lost a sister to cancer and then, just 12 hours later, his father died of a heart attack. Ariel, a second-generation Mexican American, maintained close contact with his family, particularly his mother and an older sister, who lived in an apartment in their home. Carin, of Irish descent, was closer to her father than her mother, both of whom lived out of town. Ariel's relationship with his family, which often felt intrusive to Carin, had been an ongoing source of stress in their marriage.

As for Carin's pregnancy, I was fearful for her because I knew, all too well, the course of a woman's emotional life as she carried a baby after experiencing a previous loss. This issue had come up a lot in my work with women and had also been something I had struggled with personally. In fact, I had conceived 2 months after the loss of our daughter. A previous loss, or in Carin's case, losses, coupled with the uncertainties of a subsequent pregnancy are the ingredients of an inescapable fear. I knew what my emotional limits had been, and I did not know how we would face the very possibility of another tragedy together. It was an unspeakable fear that we struggled to survive by *never* naming it.

Looking back, I think of that possibility as a "red zone," as something that we mutually felt represented a pain neither of us could have imagined survivable. It was clearly something I felt unprepared to cope with, and I often wondered, and continue to wonder, what it would have been like for us had she lost this baby. In all the therapeutic work I have done, I do not recall having feared any life circumstance in the way I feared this one. Dwelling too long on this possibility competed with my sense of "preparedness," which, in turn, threatened my image of myself as someone who could handle whatever came her way. As a general rule, relational–cultural therapy reminds us that any time we move toward an "image," we move out of engagement and toward disconnection. My only alternative, then, was to move away from this image, to ask for help, and to begin weaving a web of support for Carin and myself.

Negotiating the type of care I would provide for Carin was complex because I felt her care also included the care of her unborn child and her family. Because of this complexity, I wanted permission to engage in open communication with her obstetrician. He and I needed to be on the "same page," as the details of any complications Carin might face would help me to gauge and manage her anxiety. I asked Carin to sign a two-way consent for communication between her obstetrician and myself. Carin was not the most trusting person; she agreed, but with some reluctance and suspicion.

Carin's lack of trust would emerge as an ongoing theme in our work together. Indeed, it had been a long-term issue for her and had fueled her sense of isolation throughout her life. More recently, her baseline level of distrust had been raised considerably by her experience of betrayal by Dr. Thompson. On one hand, her lack of trust prevented her from taking in desperately needed support, while on the other hand—and paradoxically— it kept her safe from further betrayal and disappointment. This complex dynamic was the source of many of our disconnections and much of my frustration, feeling that I was not getting through to her and that she did not, or could not, trust me.

STRUGGLING FOR CONNECTION

I wish I could write that the majority of our work was done in a context of connection. In reality, we struggled with so much fear, pain, and self-blame that we seemed to make only the *occasional* connection. I longed for us to connect, for her to let herself off the hook. It just was not going to happen as long as she held onto her relentless self-blame. I also sensed I was more available in the relationship when she waived some on this is-sue. In those fleeting moments I felt like I had gotten through to her—and gained a respite from my constant feelings of ineffectiveness. As long as she blamed herself and held on to the image of herself as a failure, I was locked into an image of seeing myself as ineffective, helpless, unprepared, and even "incompetent." This was a frustrating and painful dilemma that we both felt helpless to move out of at times.

Relational–cultural theory reframes the traditional notions of "im-passe" and "resistance" as being relational in nature. Rather than looking strictly at some intrapsychic flaw (one-way thinking) in the client as the source of therapeutic failures, relational–cultural theory examines these dynamics as the products of relational disconnections or empathic fail-ures (two-way thinking). Movement out of disconnection requires looking at what both the client *and* the therapist bring to the relationship at any particular point. An examination of relational patterns is often compli-cated by our respective responses to our vulnerabilities and feelings of shame. The complexity of relational patterns is further compounded by sociopolitical influences, which are addressed in depth in the scholarship of relational–cultural theory.

Responses to shame may include that of self-blame (a belief that *I* am the problem) or other-blame (a belief that the problem is *in* the other person); intense self-blame can move a person from experiencing a relational disconnection to a more painful place described as *condemned isolation*. In this state, the person often feels completely undeserving, unlovable, and locked out of the possibility of connection. Often, individuals become self-destructive in ways that are, paradoxically, hurtful to others and to their relationships with others.

The tendency to respond to shame by other-blaming is most often indicative of power imbalances in relationships. The individual who has the most power in a relational construction, or who is working to attain or maintain the most power, typically blames the other. In the act of blaming another, the blamer has the potential to become abusive and violent, either physically, emotionally, or both. Relational–cultural theory posits that either response to shame (i.e., self- or other-blaming) leads us to a place of relational immobility. If the problem is simply in one person or the other, then the solution to averting feelings of shame is clear.

Therapists, who by most accounts carry the power in therapeutic relationships, struggle with their own shame unique to this particular role. In fact, much is written in the relational–cultural theory literature about the notion of "therapist shame." In order to examine the relational dynamics of disconnections, therapists have to engage in two-way thinking and, in a sense, give up the privilege of labeling the client as the sole source of the therapeutic disconnection as a way of managing shame. Giving up this privilege as a source of power evokes a sense of vulnerability in the therapist, particularly in those who are traditionally trained. For practitioners of relational–cultural therapy, this process is a movement toward mutuality and connection and away from shame and immobility. In fact, it is in this place of *supported vulnerability* that we find the creative energy needed to resist the sources of disconnections.

The process of developing creative means for resisting the sources of disconnections is key to developing *relational resilience*, a central goal of relational–cultural theory. During times of disconnection, it is the therapist's role to "hold" the possibility for reconnection until it can be more fully shared between the therapist and client. In a paper on relational resilience, Jordan (1992) wrote that therapists of relational–cultural theory sometimes find themselves the "lone container of hope" who have to "hold the possibility for relational resilience" (p. 6). I think these words speak to how difficult, lonely, and discouraging it can be for a therapist, whose goal is to foster relational growth through transformative connections, to find the energy and resilience to be able to do this.

In an effort to move out of our disconnections, Carin and I spent a lot of time going in circles. We talked openly about our conflicting determination and how clumsy and circular our arguments would become and about what happened to us when we got stuck. Again, traditional theories would have most likely labeled her as resistant, self-destructive, self-defeating, or worse, delusional. I have distinct memories of her sitting in front of me pregnant, sobbing, and sharing how she was "going to go to hell because there is no place in heaven for mothers who kill their babies"—as if she were unaware of being pregnant. I had such a hard time understanding the intensity of her self-blame while taking in the fact that she was going to have another baby—sooner rather than later. As stuck as we felt, things *were* going to change, and I wanted her to be ready.

Consistent with relational–cultural theory, I saw the problem as more than something that was simply *in her*; rather, it was *between us*. It was *our* disconnection that mirrored much of the isolation she felt in her life. Guided by relational–cultural theory, the question around our pattern of disconnection became, "What are *we* doing?" It would be some time before we would make sense out of our relationship. During this time we shared a sense of feeling walled off and isolated from each other. The image that comes to mind is one of her and I meeting in a prison visitation booth. The wall between us is clear yet effectively divisive. She sits on one side, I on the other. We can see each other but we are unable to touch, to reach out, to comfort, or to be comforted. In this place of meeting we always hope for a connection, then we notice the darkness. We struggle to connect while feeling bogged down by a context we cannot escape. We wish we were anywhere else.

As a prisoner, Carin beckons me to come and meet with her. My job is to escort her out of that place, that debilitating emotional hell. Before I can walk her out of her prison, however, she needs me to help her see Noah's life and death more clearly. Indeed there are many things Carin cannot see clearly. Not only can she not see Noah's death clearly, she cannot see herself and *all* of who she is or all of who she will become. I will soon learn just how bad she needs clarity on many issues and what she will do with the facts when they do not fit with her image of herself as a bad, unlovable, unworthy, and condemned mother who failed to protect her son from his untimely demise. I would also come to understand what would happen to me when my time with her did not reinforce my image of myself as a competent, trustworthy, patient, effective, and creative therapist.

PLAYING OUT THE PARADOX

As the months passed, it became clear that her pregnancy was viable. Much of our early work included managing her grief and the anxieties regarding level II ultra sounds, genetic testing, and other blood work. Although all the results were encouraging, there was an increased chance that she could have another baby with birth defects, given Noah's history. But what *was* Noah's history? What exactly had been the cause of all of his problems? Up to this point we had had no answers. The autopsy report had not been sent to the pediatrician, and the only evidence that seemed to matter to Carin was the stained blanket, which she kept hidden.

One day Carin called, unable to contain her need to know the results of Noah's autopsy. She had grown increasingly anxious and was now very upset that the pediatrician's office was not being more aggressive in obtaining the report. Because Carin was so emotionally debilitated, I chose to intervene by calling the coroner's office myself. It was not long before I spoke with the examining physician who shared the details of her findings with me.

I called Carin back, anticipating a well-deserved breakthrough, because the autopsy results would finally provide her with concrete evidence disputing a simple suffocation. She answered the phone, terrified, almost panicked, yet desperate to hear what had been found. "Frontal lobe nodes," I shared. "He had nodes in his frontal lobe, Carin. They are like little tumors and were the cause of a catastrophic seizure, the cause of his death." The coroner had been very understanding and volunteered to speak with her personally.

After a moment of silence Carin began to question the intent of the results. Her response was not one of relief but of suspicion. "People are probably telling me this just to protect me," she insisted. I was struck with how unbelievable her doubt was and I remember asking something like: "Are you saying that you think that your therapist and the coroner and the pediatrician and the examining doctor in the ER and your obstetrician all got together to conspire a story to save you from the fact that you killed your son? Is that what you believe?" "Yes," she replied.

I felt a lot of things in that moment. I was stunned, disappointed, and even angry. On the other hand, I got, for the first time, how "locked up" and frightened she was. I knew I *had* to figure out a way to be empathic with her feelings—and at that point in time, I felt very discouraged about how I was going to do so. I was reminded that the biggest challenge to working in this model is being empathic with the "other side of the paradox." In other words, it is easy to be with Carin's grief and her "need to know." It is during those times that I am more active in the relationship with her and that we work toward connection. Then, just when we have an opportunity for a moment of clarity, she turns away out of fear and, once again, we are left feeling isolated and cut off from each other.

The hardest part was working to stay empathic with her fear when I did not understand how it was protecting her. Understanding the role of her fear was a very important piece of the work, and it would be some time before we would make any sense of it. I did not know how we ever would. I also needed to be empathic with my own frustration and sense of shame over not being able to find a way to connect with her. After all, I was the therapist who was supposed to be able to hold the possibility for connection when things got rough. Every time I doubted myself, I would feel the shame again and, after all, I had a "hot button" for feeling incompetent.

Again and again, Carin beckons me to meet her in the visitation booth long enough for me to give her a glimpse of what life could be like. I offer to lead her out, walk with her, hold her hand, even carry her on my back, and each time she refuses and retreats back to her cell. Sometimes in response I pound on the glass wall, scream for her to make a move, to let herself out, and each time she is unable to move. During these times I struggle with an image much like the one that has condemned Carin: that I am ineffective, a failure, and that no matter what I do or how hard I work, and I *am* willing and wanting to work, I will lose her, just like she lost Noah. At my worst I feel afraid, immobile, ashamed, and like a failure. And I know that Carin feels this way most of the time.

My resilience in this relationship had everything to do with my own self-empathy and my ability to keep my work with Carin and my feelings in context. I was challenged to be compassionate with my own history and traditional training. Traditionally trained therapists are taught to leave their lives at the door when they enter a session, but aspects of my life are as much of who I am as my right hand—neither of which are going to be left anywhere. I had learned in my own therapy that I could not run circles around my pain, and now it was time to stop running circles around Carin's pain.

Looking back, it seems the answers to some of the questions I had neglected to ask were now taking shape. How would our shared experiences impact our relationship and our mutual growth? Clearly, one of my vulnerabilities, in spite of my "preparedness," was that I simply had a hard time tolerating anyone feeling that kind of debilitating pain. I also knew that so much of my own healing had come from the willingness of others to be with me in my pain. My dogged determination to impact Carin's experience, combined with an acknowledgment of what my own needs had been, enabled me to "sit" with her in her prison instead of doing all I could to lead her out.

DETERMINATION

In spite of the autopsy results, Carin was determined to blame herself. Now that Noah had been diagnosed with brain anomalies, she insisted that she must have caused that too. "I know it must have happened when I got kicked in the stomach catching Benjamin when he jumped into the pool," she explained. It seemed, in spite of all my efforts, she was determined to take full responsibility for Noah's death, and now his health problems as well. She began to beat herself up regarding the medical interventions to which she had consented. She should have been with him more. She should have noticed his color. She believed she had missed something, and because of her "neglect," she had exacerbated his declining health.

Over time, Carin became increasingly anxious, and she began to call between sessions. I always responded to Carin's calls, and I never discouraged her from calling. One aspect of developing self-empathy occurs through an authentic experience of *all* of who we are. If my goal was to have her bring more and more of herself into our relationship—which, at this time, was more of her anxiety—then I needed to make room for it through my responsiveness. I had given up my need to "fix it" for her by pulling her out of her experience, deciding that if she were "stuck in jail," at least she did not have to be there alone. It seemed that the more present we were with her emotional experience, the more engaged she became in the physical experience of her pregnancy.

Eventually, her anxiety shifted. Her calls began to involve questions regarding the health of her unborn baby, which I considered progress. By now she knew she was pregnant with a boy, a very active baby boy. When he would sleep she would worry, and when he was awake, any normal flips, twists, or rolls became suspect. We had all anticipated this kind of obsessive focus. In fact, early on there was some discussion of a planned Cesarean section in order to spare Carin (and Ariel) the potential for any traumatic response that might be evoked during labor and delivery. We would soon learn that Carin's traumatic triggers would come much earlier.

For the moment, Ariel seemed set on a planned Cesarean section, and I worried about how the seeming lack of trust in Carin's body to do what it needed to do for a vaginal delivery might impact her mental health. After all, Meg had died in utero as a result of a cord accident. At this point her obstetrician was willing to take "the path of the least anxieties," even after stressing the benefits of a vaginal birth.

When Carin reached the point of fetal survivability in her pregnancy (our initial marker was 28 weeks), things shifted again. Continuing to carry the baby, now that he could theoretically survive outside of her body, became almost intolerable to her. Most women fear delivering at this stage, but for Carin, the idea of carrying him any longer than she had to was overwhelming. In a sense, this milestone was a source of trauma.

Once again, I needed help, so I called a friend of mine who was a certified birth doula, someone else I knew quite well.

The doula, whom I will call Katy, had helped ground me in my body when I became pregnant after losing Samantha. Katy herself had also suffered the loss of a daughter, who was stillborn at full term. I felt her experiences would give her a jump-start in establishing a relationship with Carin. Indeed, Carin did learn to trust Katy, and it was comforting for me to be able to consult on certain aspects of Carin's care with yet another professional. Katy took a very direct approach with Carin. When Carin would start complaining she was ready to deliver, Katy would firmly ask: "What is your goal? If your goal is to have a healthy baby you can take home after delivery, you do not want to have him now." Slowly, Carin, in spite of her fear, became more comfortable with her pregnancy and set milestones for herself that helped her in carrying the baby to term.

By my making room in our relationship for her fear, Carin slowly felt less of it as she became more grounded in the idea that her baby's development was on an upward spiral and that every hour mattered. She grew more comfortable with the idea of going into labor on her own, and she gradually began to look forward to the birth of her son. We wondered together what it might be like for something wonderful to happen to her. Talking about this was almost as difficult as it was to talk about the possibility of another possible loss.

In some ways, Carin seemed afraid for *anything* to happen. We often laughed about how much she wanted him here but wanted nothing to do with getting him here. Yet, in the end, Carin gave birth to a healthy 10.6-pound baby boy, "Nathan." We took a respite from therapy so that she could heal and adjust to the demands of nursing and infant care. I believed that Nathan's arrival would be a huge relief for Carin, and I looked forward to our work taking a different course.

SHAMEFUL DISCLOSURES

When Nathan was about 2 months old, Carin called needing a letter supporting her application for disability benefits. The social worker processing her request indicated that he wanted me to address her diagnoses and the reason why she was not on any medication, if she were doing so poorly. I wrote a letter highlighting the various aspects of her mental health status and explained, in great detail, the benefits that nursing had on the physical and mental health of both mother and baby. After a short time she received a letter indicating that her request for social security benefits had been approved.

Carin did not know when she would start receiving financial support. When she pursued clarification on the issue with the local social security office, she was given the runaround. The ambiguity became a serious concern for Carin and sent her into a downward spiral like none other I had seen in her. The calls resumed, as did our therapy. Carin was becoming increasingly anxious again, even paranoid. She was convinced she was being "investigated" and that the social security office now knew she had a new baby for whom she was unable to care. She was desperately afraid that someone would simply knock on her door and take her kids away. Once again, she was a prisoner in her own home. She avoided going out and would not even walk by the windows in her house; she was particularly afraid of the police, and on one particularly bad day she called me, literally unable to leave her bedroom.

In spite of all our new issues, our work did take an unexpected turn. To my astonishment, Carin confessed to having had the need to believe that she had caused Noah's death, because she could not have survived her pregnancy with Nathan thinking that Noah's health problems may have been something genetic, or something beyond her control that could repeat itself. It seemed so simple. Her strategy for disconnection was now named a *strategy for survival* that had been essential to her well-being during her pregnancy. Holding on to the belief that she had caused Noah's health problems *and* his subsequent death kept her from going to yet another place of intolerable vulnerability.

The impact of this mutual understanding was one of the most powerful moments in our work together. I was deeply moved, and I acknowledged how hard it must have been for her to have me work so hard to talk her out of exactly what she was needing to do to survive. We have revisited this issue on many occasions. Carin told me that it would have been devastating for her had I taken any other approach. Paradoxically, she needed me to believe in her as much as she needed to blame herself. Understanding this has helped me grow more comfortable with all of the uncertainties in this work. I have learned that being stuck, even in a seemingly dangerous place, is sometimes exactly where we need to be.

Relational–cultural theory posits that therapists can work to co-create moments of healing in therapy through an authentic responsiveness that demonstrates how we are impacted by our clients' experiences. In essence, moments of healing are created when our clients "take in," or are empathic with, our experience of them. This is a complex, bidirectional process that relational–cultural theory refers to as the flow of *mutual empathy*. The role of mutual empathy in my relationship with Carin stemmed from my willingness to "sit" with her fear. We participated in a mutual exercise of respect for something that, at times, seemed to grow out of control. Once

Carin sensed my deep respect for her fear, she was able to bring even more of herself into our relationship.

During one session, I noticed Carin working hard not to avert her eyes. It seemed she was mustering up some courage, and after some time she stated, "I need to share something with you, and I know you're going to think I'm crazy. I haven't even told my husband this, and I'm not sure I want him to know." She went on to tell me that since she was a young child she had lived a sort of fantasy life. Through the years she had spent countless hours living in an imaginary world as a way to cope with the isolation and stressors in her life. She even suggested that I watch the movie *Passion of Mind* with Demi Moore, which I did. I thought it captured her experience quite well, and we talked about it for a long time.

It all started when she was 12, about the time her parents divorced. At first, she would just sit down and "write a story" in her head, construct another life. Over the years the characters became more real to her and she had come to actively converse with the various "players." In fact, it had become so out of control that her now 3-year-old son Benjamin had recently asked to whom she was talking. She shared that because she had been feeling so anxious, she had increasingly indulged in this behavior as a way of coping. She expressed feeling out of control, incredibly frightened, and deeply ashamed. To this day she reminds me to appreciate how hard it was for her to share this aspect of herself.

I was, in fact, deeply moved that she was able to share this with me, and I remind her of this from time to time. I was amazed how she had concocted such a brilliant, creative way of coping. When she worried that she was really crazy, I reminded her that she could be drinking alcohol, abusing drugs, or doing any of a million other things that people do who are very self-destructive. Yet for Carin, this inner life *was* self-destructive. It was a strategy for disconnection that kept her from relating authentically to the "real" people in her life. Instead of putting her feelings into her relationships, she would silence herself, move to a place of condemned isolation, and connect with her imaginary support system. When she would get angry with Ariel, for example, she simply turned to her imaginary backup husband, who understood her and accepted her for all of who she was.

This fantasy world had become a prison from which Carin wanted out—and, indeed, she found the courage and strength in our relationship to leave. Shortly after this session Carin told Ariel her secret. She was no longer alone in her secret, shameful life. Ariel was incredibly responsive and much of the tension in their marriage simply deflated. This experience was empowering for Carin, and it marked the beginning of changes in the way she participated in many of her relationships.

CONCLUSION

One of the most painful areas of growth for me in my relationship with Carin was learning to manage the sense of helplessness that fueled an incredible surge of negative images of myself as an ineffective therapist. Resisting these images meant opening myself up to new images of myself as a therapist who could be both vulnerable *and* strong. This experience had multiple layers of meaning and taught me many lessons about courage, strength, and resilience.

One of the simple truths about this complicated relationship was that I, too, had experienced a loss. Although we shared a mutual understanding of some aspects of this experience, I was always aware of how different we were. I learned that even around similarities, and maybe even *especially* around similarities, therapists need to be exceptionally attentive. If not, we fail to ask the right kinds of questions, if we think to ask them at all. The scholars of relational–cultural theory have always reminded us to work toward creating a therapeutic environment, and such an environment is about learning, not knowing. I guess I would say that my "knowing," in this case, had the potential to get in the way of my understanding and tolerating Carin's experience.

Being empathic with my own paradoxical responses enabled me to work to restore and hold the possibility of connection and to move out of what could have been mutual and chronic isolation and shame. Just as I had to make more and more room for Carin's feelings, I had to do the same for my own feelings of helplessness and shame. I often made a point to remember that the simple fact of our being together was an act of reaching, a yearning in motion. In essence, our "being together" was, in and of itself, both a mark and a source of mutual resilience. I think this perspective captures what many find so powerful about relational–cultural theory, which, in my opinion, is in and of itself, a powerful source of resilience against many destructive factors.

In the end it was Carin who, in spite of her suspicion and mistrust, taught me about trust, honesty, and how to ask for help—something I will always work to get better at and do more of. Asking for help and clarity means we have to acknowledge our vulnerabilities as therapists. In short, I believe that misusing, abusing, or simply relying on diagnostic labels is one of the ways that therapists resist their vulnerabilities to feeling ineffective, helpless, or incompetent. When things do not move in therapy, we have the privilege to blame it on this "disorder" that is wrong with our client. In doing so, we gain control of our feelings by naming where, and in whom, the problem lies. At the same time we deplete our creativity and dismantle the context of our clients' lives.

All told, Carin suffered from a complicated mix of grief, loss, PTSD, a garden variety of depression (major and postpartum, several times over), betrayal, isolation, yearning, sensitivity, hormones, normal pregnancy neurosis, shame, sleep deprivation, secrets, paranoia, imagination, a mother's love, and a broken heart. In all honestly, I sometimes wished for an encompassing diagnosis that would have neatly fit together the pieces of Carin's experience. Overall, however, such a diagnosis was not central to my thinking.

I will always work to get better at understanding the strategies we all exercise to protect our emotional vulnerabilities, whatever the context. In the meantime, I look forward to living more questions with Carin—with the exception, of course, of the question of what happened to Noah. For now, we have dueling stories. We probably always will.

REFERENCE

Jordan, J. V. (1992). Relational resilience. *Work in Progress, No. 57*. Wellesley, MA: Stone Center Working Paper Series.

Part III

Applications to Couple, Family, and Group Therapy

Psychotherapy is often utilized as a forum for the exploration of relational systems. Although the central concepts of relational–cultural theory remain the same for both individual and systems therapy, there are certain differences and complexities that merit examination. In individual therapy, the only "in vivo" relationship is that of the therapist and client, and the larger context of relational systems, such as culture and family of origin, is experienced and understood through the vehicle of this relationship. When the therapist is sitting face to face with an existing system of relationships, he or she not only becomes part of that system but also observes and intermittently joins the multitude of subsystems that exist within it. In treatment with systems larger than the therapist–client dyad, there are multiple and changing levels of relational connections and disconnections that call for recognition. For example, a group therapy context may contain within it seven or eight individuals with different central relational paradoxes, as well as various group subsystems, each with its own central relational paradox. Family systems may, at times, consist of two relational groups—that of the parent or parents and that of the sibling subset—each with its own strategies of disconnection, relational images, and the like. In these cases, the relational systems themselves are the locus of treatment, with individual transformation as an artifact of the larger systemic changes. A significant opportunity that is afforded by working with relational systems, furthermore, is that of observing and becoming a part of the continuous shift in power relations and the sharing of expertise with all members of the system. Fluid expertise forms an essential mechanism for relational change in these contexts.

The chapters in this section examine the practice of psychotherapy within various relational systems. Each of the four case examples is a unique type of system that is also singular in the particular relational issues that emerge, their cultural contexts and attendant controlling images, the negotiation of differences, the therapist's place within each system, and the evolution of power in these relationships. In each case, the therapist effectively highlights her own contributions to the relational processes as well as her personal conduits for empathic connection.

Cindy Walls's work with a white lesbian couple whose relationship is complicated not only by their marginalized status as lesbians, but also by issues of clinical depression and early trauma, reveals much about the delicate negotiation of relational intimacy against a powerful backdrop of disconnecting forces. The significant emphasis on engaging and increasing the capacity for mutual empathy in the face of vulnerability highlights its centrality as a mechanism for decreasing power abuse and deepening connection.

Karen Skerrett's case with a white, heterosexual, married couple reveals a somewhat different set of relational images and dynamics, in which issues of class, gender, and relational competition are paramount. Skerrett emphasizes an increased awareness of the relationship between these individuals and its treatment as a third, and in many ways, primary, entity in need of empathic attention. She defines her own role as, among other things, the guardian of this "we" and experiences herself as in a relationship with their relationship.

Family therapy is the focus of Roseann Adams's case. At the core of this therapy is the factor of cross-cultural difference: that of a black family working with a white therapist. The crisis of differences that emerges within the family itself and the arduous task of creating and sustaining a newly blended family are at the center of the work. Adams's own relational images are both powerful contributors to, and informants of, the complexity of relational processes within the system as a whole and its many subsystems. Additionally, this therapy represents an example of a prescribed short-term managed care case and thus speaks to the limitations and possibilities inherent in a relational–cultural approach within this context.

Nikki Fedele presents a case example of a group therapy and focuses, in particular, on a dyadic subsystem that forms within it. One dynamic within groups is the function of roles as strategies of disconnection from the group as a whole. Such roles are based largely on the individual relational images brought to the group experience. In this regard, the group can be seen as a microcosm of the range of relational contexts in which all people must function, such as sibling and parent, family and community, and so on. It is a particularly complex task for the therapist, as both participant and observer, as Fedele's experience within the group effectively highlights.

All of the following case examples illustrate the overarching principles inherent in relational–cultural therapy. The core assumption, as suggested in Chapter 1, is that people grow through action in relationship. These cases are attempts to answer the central question of how the therapy relationship can contribute to, and strengthen, the capacity for resilience and empowering movement in connection.

7

Me, Them, Us
Developing Mutuality
in a Couple's Therapy

CYNTHIA WALLS

*R*elational awareness, being in relational flow, authenticity, and mutuality and the transformations of disconnections are processes to which many couple therapists are acutely attuned and work hard to help their client couples achieve. Couple therapists know that when people are involved in mutual, growth-enhancing relationships, they feel vital, and that vitality inoculates them against the anxieties, depressions, and despair born out of isolation. And we all know that when relationships go awry, life can feel oppressive and difficult to navigate. Accordingly, much of the current research and practice in the couple therapy field has focused on the necessity to build or shore up (ever-elusive) intimacy in couples (Gottman & Silver, 2000; Pinsof, 2000; Real, 2002; Schnarch, 1997).

Susan Johnson, a marital therapist and the developer of emotionally focused therapy, states that the focus of a couple's treatment is to "address attachment concerns, reduce insecurities, and foster creation of a secure bond. The main issues are connection and disconnection, separateness and closeness" (Johnson, 1996, p. 21). This view represents a shift away from past theories that dominated the family therapy field, with their emphasis on separation, individuation, and boundary articulation. More and more, couple therapists strive to help their clients achieve a greater capacity for intimacy. This term, *intimacy*, used frequently in the couple therapy field yet ever difficult to operationalize, is similar to what relational–cultural theory refers to as *mutuality*. Unfortunately, mutuality suffers from the same problem of definitional clarity; for mutuality, like intimacy, is a process best understood by its experience rather than by its description. You know you are in it by how you feel. Intimacy and mutuality are not commodities nor constant states, but processes one moves in and out of and recognizes by how it feels. Mutuality follows a developmental course that appropriately unfolds as certain tests are met: Is the person trustworthy? Is he or she able to be sensitive and responsive? Are the relational images held by each person optimistic and flexible enough so that empathic responses can be anticipated and asked for, and the inevitable experiences of empathic failure can be weathered? With time, hopefully, there is a gradual deepening of the connection. But relationships can stall, maintaining a disconnected or conflictive holding pattern in the testing zone, and never quite make it over the threshold. These are the relationships many couples bring to treatment.

Helping to move relationships toward connection is one of the many common areas of focus between relational–cultural theory and couple treatment. Both attend to the intricacies of connection and intimate space, and to the facilitative or destructive processes within that space. The couple therapist is trained to focus on the relationship in the room—first the relationship of the two patients, and then, between the therapist and patients. Couple work can require from the therapist both a higher level of activity, and, conversely, a deliberate remove in the effort to help two people bring themselves to each other, to talk to each other, often when they have been struggling with each other for years. How much easier it can be just to have one patient tell the therapist about the problem, bypassing his or her partner, who, if present, might derail the opening-up process by interrupting, blaming, and criticizing. But it is precisely this problematic interaction that needs to become the focus of couple treatment. The challenge for the therapist is to know when to move in and when to move out. Certainly, it is important to intercede by helping couples talk to each other *through* the therapist when they are embroiled in a troublesome interaction, unable to truly hear what the other is saying, particularly when the interaction has the potential to create further disconnection. Just as significantly, however, it is important to let them struggle with each other, within a manageable range of frustration, to find their own route toward better connection, through which they create something new together—a template for mutuality.

Many couple therapists describe experiencing themselves in the alternating social roles of participant and observer, trying to orchestrate something between the couple, functioning at times more like an educator or a

coach, or, at worst, a referee. This is not to say that attention to the therapeutic alliance (the relationship between therapist and couple) is not essential, valued, or cultivated. No kind of therapy can take place without
connection between all involved. But the relationship between the couple
and the couple's therapist is most often "less intense" than between an individual and the individual's therapist, as it would naturally be in any context when one moves from the intimacy of the dyad to the complexity of
the multiple. Johnson writes: "the intensity is mediated in marital therapy
by the presence of probably the most important attachment figure in each
individual's life, the other partner" (1996, p. 36).

Accordingly, with some of these differences in focus and action, it
can be easier for the couple's therapist to hide, to minimize his or her
own importance, except as a catalyst for the couple. Indeed, the couple's
therapist may maintain that the real intimacy being built is between these
"other two," and any problem in the relationships in the room is about
them and their difficulties. But where, exactly, does that view leave us, as
couple therapists, in this process? How can we help couples achieve a
greater level of intimacy/mutuality and a relational awareness so that
their disconnections can be transformed more efficiently and effectively
if we do not model these processes ourselves? If, in our job as couple therapists, we ask our clients to take risks with each other and us, to be more
open and more vulnerable, then we ourselves cannot hold back in these
endeavors. Mutuality is at its best when we "put our money where our
mouth is"—when we, the therapists, stretch ourselves to grow in ways that
we are asking clients to grow. We are asked not to work "on" our clients'
problems, but to work "in" them—to bring ourselves to the therapy more
fully, to be authentic in our presence, and to strive for mutuality in the
process.

INTRODUCING JAN AND RAMONA

Jan and Ramona showed up in my office about 5 years ago on the recommendation of Jan's individual therapist. They are a white, lesbian couple
in their 40s. Jan is small, athletic, wiry, and intense. She grabs attention
and can fill a room with her energy and emotion. Ramona has a quieter
demeanor. She is petite, soft, thoughtful, and somewhat retiring. Her
presence, although understated, is equally strong, but in a manner that
inches up on others, rather than meeting them full force. Both women are
bright, involved, and accomplished professionals: Jan is a therapist and
Ramona is a writer. They have been together for 13 years, living together
for 11 of them.

Over the past couple of years, as their attachment developed and their professional lives settled, and as they were both well established in a good course of individual therapy, they began to bring more of themselves into the relationship. Ramona's longstanding clinical depression had finally been treated with successful individual psychotherapy and medication, and she was beginning to move out of her retreat and to want more for herself and from Jan. This shift was not an entirely positive experience for Ramona, because expanding her needs produced numerous fears.

Ramona had grown up in a family with whom she struggled, usually unsuccessfully, to feel noticed and to maintain a sense of her own importance. The emotional availability of her parents (particularly her mother) felt inconsistent, and she learned rather quickly that the best adaptation to disappointment of her needs was not to need openly. She made herself scarce. Overall, it was best to keep things to herself, both pain and excitement. She paints many vivid images of her earlier existence, consisting mainly of feeling banished; later, she opted to retreat prophylactically. As we got to know each other better, she would describe some of these memories. Sad images of feeling very alone, tearful, and off by herself were commonplace. Alternately, she remembered how she fought intensely to be recognized in the family, especially by her mother, as she moved into an emboldened adolescence. Her clamor was met with an even stronger rejection, and Ramona eventually retreated in demoralized resignation. She left home while still in high school to live with another relative, as the discord between her and her mother became too great. They had been, and still are, unable to reach each other in significant ways. Reinforcing this disconnection is her mother's response to Ramona's lesbianism, which she also struggled to represent to her mother, and, to this day, has to "remind" her mother at each visit "who" she is. Bringing Jan along on the trips home is a reminder, and her mother's rejection of Jan is the continual evidence that Ramona is not welcomed for who she is, for her needs and desires.

Jan, through her own individual therapy, was beginning to move into aspects of her life that had long been secreted away. They, too, felt incredibly unsafe to bring forward. Jan describes a fairly unremarkable upbringing, growing up in a family in which she felt loved and attended to, but primarily in response to those aspects of herself which were considered strong, capable, and entertaining. What stood out in her history were notable experiences of trauma. Beginning at the age of 4, she was diagnosed with a genitourinary problem. Treatment for this condition required numerous procedures over a span of several years, beginning with several courses involving dilation of her vaginal and urethral areas, when, as she remembers it, metal instruments were "stuck up her." These procedures were all done in a military hospital with negligible, to no, anesthesia.

Eventually surgery was done to correct the problem, but it was followed by several more dilation procedures. She was "finished" with all the procedures and treatment for her condition by the age of 8. She remembers these procedures as being excruciatingly painful, in response to which she would eventually dissociate and not remember her body from the "head down." She recalled that she had to be a "big girl" and not to squirm or cry for the benefit of the hospital personnel and her distraught mother, who would stand beside her, holding her hand. Added to her having to endure unbearable physical pain was the emotional trauma of feeling that her fears and need for comfort (or rescue) were not acceptable. After all, this was a necessary, certified medical procedure, done by caring, professional staff.

Judith Herman (1992) and Alice Miller (1981) write separately that the hallmark of psychological trauma is not just the experience of the traumatic event itself, but also the lack of empathic response to the feelings of the trauma victim. If there were a guiding relational principle in operation for Jan during these childhood years, it was that this basic human need to be taken care of and responded to, when feeling afraid, small, and vulnerable, was filled with shame. Adding tenfold to this difficult, isolating feeling is the fact that the medical procedures she endured have a pronounced presence in her sexual fantasy life. The surgery and her sexual life have become encapsulated in trauma-ridden fantasies (essentially replays of the procedures), leaving her with feelings of extreme self-disgust and immense humiliation. To her these fantasies indicate how loathsome and depraved she is; she believes that, if others knew about them, they would feel compelled to leave her. This need for concealment—for shrouding aspects of herself in secrecy—has also been reinforced mightily by our culture. Being lesbian had produced a very real need to hide, to feel ashamed of her desires, and to be unable to represent herself fully. As a result, she has overdeveloped strategies of disconnection, as does Ramona. Now, in the relationship with Ramona, anxiety about her sexual needs and the prospect of placing herself in defenseless, dependent states is more than she can manage. This desire to be cared for, especially in vulnerable, shame-filled places, was greatly compromised by the traumatic events—which is why she learned to hide it. She also had a father and mother who encouraged her "tough-as-nails" stance and who either ignored or openly discouraged signs of weakness. She could give to, and need openly from, others, but she primarily felt good only about her strong, compassionate, competent self. She could be recognized and lauded for how good and tough she was; the weak and afraid was hidden away.

These old relational images led both Jan and Ramona to a sense that to openly represent themselves and to need others was, at best, unwarranted, or, at worst, emotionally dangerous (causing shame, humiliation, desertion). They learned many ways to hide their desires and developed various strategies of disconnection. It became a cruel irony: Their efforts to protect themselves only made matters worse, and their attempts to deal with the shame, depression, and anxiety only intensified their discomfort. Jan's dominant relational image dictated that showing certain forms of weakness, particularly fear, would be seen as "bad" and lead to her desertion. Ramona's relational images advanced her belief that, if she were too expressive of her needs, revealed too much excitement and desire, she would be seen as "bad"—which, in turn, would be met with harsh disapproval and potential abandonment. They both feared some form of desertion, and their attempts to protect against it led to its counterpart, estrangement.

This was the point at which they had come to see me. They were afraid that their relationship was not going to make it. The periods of disengagement had resulted in feelings of isolation and a growing stagnation in their connection. The relationship was not providing much sustenance for either of them. Often their attempts at engagement were fraught with anxiety, leading to fairly predictable conflict, and ending in helpless resignation. Frequently, as relationships deepen and intimate longings are felt, things do not go smoothly. Contrary to romantic notions, the deepening of attachments is not primarily a blissful time for most couples, unless both persons have been blessed with a history of consistent responsiveness to each of their needs. Particularly, if one or both persons have a history of trauma or other extreme disconnection, closeness can feel frightening, as it threatens to disarm the long entrenched efforts toward self-protection. As the attachment strengthens and relational images surface, old, familiar, and troubling ways of feeling often get stimulated, creating fears about getting close. Intense anxiety or depression may ensue.

Opening up, getting a glimpse of new ways of being, and exposing long-hidden aspects of themselves were creating a tremendous amount of fear in both Jan and Ramona. By virtue of their individual growth, they were straining the limits of the relationship that they had tacitly erected over the years, based on the premise that to be "close" meant keeping aspects of themselves far away, out of connection. They had enacted their own relational paradox: In order to be in relationship with each other, they had to keep certain aspects out of the interaction. The desire to be known was matched by the fear of being known.

BEGINNING THE THERAPY

As I had heard about them from their individual therapists, I felt prepared for Jan to be extremely reluctant, anxious, and fearful, and that she would manage these feelings by going on the offensive. She did all that. In the first session she could barely stay in the room. She wanted to leave after half an hour, and then insisted they only come every other week. Her anxiety was palpable and left me feeling scared; it succeeded, though, in pulling me in—there was something potent underneath, something to which I could relate. In the first several weeks, I lived with a fairly steady concern that I would be unable to reach her, and if I did, that I would probably disappoint her. She did not fail to let me know when that had occurred. Our beginning sessions were punctuated with retorts, such as, "That was stupid," in response to a comment of mine, or, at best, a warning, "Now don't say anything stupid"—which I never seemed successful at heeding. During this early phase of the therapy, I felt moderately to acutely self-conscious, bumbling, and silently afraid—alternately fearful that I would lose them or that I would not. Jan, at times, tried her hardest to beat me back, but she was simultaneously able to engage me. There was a humor, toughness, and vivacity about her that always stood fast, and I grew to admire and enjoy her. Additionally, this rocky beginning was given some grounding by a tenacity on my part, born out of my relational images. In this case, I was overly determined not to be dismissed. Old, painful experiences in my own family around abandonment have often led me into struggles in this realm. I am never quite sure about whether to stay in there and fight for the connection, or to retreat in protection from the anticipated rejection. This moving toward/moving away would be a constant pattern in our relationship: Jan would be angrily dismissive, and I would feel challenged to "hang in there." My struggle around whether to leave Jan alone and wind up alone myself versus pursuing her was the heart of the therapy. In a different way, I struggled with Ramona as well. When a therapist struggles with a client's core dynamics, which interface so well with the therapist's own, there are opportunities either for hiding or for authenticity. Authenticity does not require disclosure or even exposure, necessarily. Authenticity does mean that the "therapist tries to be with the thoughts and feelings occurring in the relationship. It also means that the therapist tries to be with the movement towards connection, the fears of that movement, and the strategies of disconnection" (Miller, 1999, p. 2). There was an opportunity. I opted for hiding. It was an old, familiar attempt to control my anxiety.

Week after week, as I heard the outer door to my office open upon Jan and Ramona's arrival for our appointment and felt my anxiety, I would take a deep breath, try to still the churning, and steel myself against its intrusion—lest the anxiety overwhelm me and become apparent to them. Initially, I did not give much thought to why I was anxious, unfortunately. I did not engage in much reflection. Rather, the anxiety was something to dispose of, quickly, and mainly through denial or a counter-phobic determination to plow ahead. I kept what I was experiencing largely hidden (I thought). I felt a lot, but did not know much, about my own reactions and theirs. As I endured this experience of disconnection over several sessions, a vague knowing began to unfold within me. The anxiety was familiar. It was in reaction to, or in anticipation of, feeling dismissed. In my old mode of adaptation I would either retreat in response to feeling rejected or stay in there, quietly, off to the side, but very aware, waiting for the other to come forward. Fortunately, the latter is not a bad tack for a therapist to take. Soon Jan and Ramona's tales would unfold.

In addition to my crude strategies of disconnection, I was additionally fortified with the belief that Jan's anger was "defensive," and with the fact that Ramona fairly quickly established herself as my ally. Where Jan was taut and prickly, Ramona was soft and flexible. I felt I had a wide berth with her; she would give me a lot of leeway, not demand much, and generally be pleased with what I had to offer. From early on, with little discouragement from me, Ramona adopted an informal cotherapist position. She helped Jan and I find a way to each other, often serving as interpreter as well as enforcer, fixing Jan with a soft, though firm, look when she threatened to bolt. She consistently was the one to start the sessions, bringing forward significant incidents and interactions from the week, expressing both her concerns and letting me know what Jan was experiencing, when Jan was reluctant to articulate it. "Jan has something she wants to talk about," was a common refrain, and Ramona would proceed to gently prod her forward. She also made sure they came back week after week, in the face of Jan's high anxiety. She held a firm resolve, which I learned to appreciate. Her ability to persevere in the relationship and in the therapy was notable. She was not going to be denied. When it later became apparent, her particular role, positioned "off to the side," and the unconscious collaboration with me on its development raised some troubling concerns. It was a position that kept her out of the fray, allowing her to advance her needs through a side door, by way of Jan. Ramona was able to camouflage her excitement and pace her desire to be known. I tacitly supported this maneuver, for besides her help in the interpreter/enforcer role, she was a deeper, more personally felt ally for me. Ramona could "spell" me in my emotionally fraught efforts to stay in there with Jan while feeling pushed back. She provided a camaraderie I had not realized how much I had sorely missed. Unbeknown to all of us, for awhile, Ramona's and my collaboration was creating an old, uncomfortable feeling for Jan. Ramona and I had become a "professional team," which Jan later would describe as creating more discomfort than support. Understandably, this collusion evoked painful associations to her surgeries.

As it became clear, in the weeks ahead, that we would keep each other and that the therapy was a "go," I established myself in a fairly comfortable role as the "expert," helping them with themselves, their problems, and their relationship. It is a position that provides a certain observatory distance, and it is one I often slide into at the beginning of a therapy, particularly when I am feeling unnerved. The distancing of the expert role helps me to mediate the uncertainty about my potential helpfulness and allows me to affirm myself as someone who has an expertise and from whom they can get something of value in their effort to improve the relationship.

We all took a step back, I exhaled, and we brought our collective heads together to try to figure out what was going on: "What were they needing help with? What were they experiencing?" Enlisting the couple in a "let's tackle this together" mode, in an attempt to diffuse the usual counterblaming sequences, is often a helpful first move and establishes a tone of collaboration, which can be hard to come by with a conflictual couple (Bergman & Surrey, 1992). I had enough equanimity at this point to reflect on what I saw in front of me and to attend to my reactions, as they did theirs, and we embarked on a fairly typical couple's therapy course, trying to understand their conflict and seek ways to repair the resulting disengagement.

TOWARD MUTUAL EMPATHY THROUGH FEAR

Moving forward involved engaging the identified stress at the level they were able to articulate it. Initially, this entailed honoring their strategies of disconnection (Miller, 1999). The work of familiarizing ourselves with the disconnections and respecting and appreciating the fears that caused them was an important launching point. Of what were they afraid? Jan readily identified being afraid *for* Ramona. She could spend the greater part of the initial sessions describing, with intense fretfulness, her worry about Ramona's lack of productivity with her writing. Ramona could stay holed up in her office writing for days at a time, but when Jan would pass by, she always seemed to catch her at the times when Ramona was resting on the couch or playing solitaire on the computer, instead of writing. Catastrophic fears abounded that Ramona would become increasingly depressed and dissolute, and eventually spiral down into some horrible state, lose her livelihood, all respect, and be left with nothing but her own self-disgust. Jan felt she had to maintain a prodding vigilance, lest Ramona "not get anything done" and "circle the drain." Not surprisingly, Ramona complained that Jan "would not leave her alone" and trust her to get done whatever was needed. Ramona felt scrutinized, pestered, and criticized, in a manner that made her want to retreat even more from both her work and Jan, and which compounded her already demoralized and fatigued state. Of course, Ramona's response only exacerbated Jan's anxiety and led to the very disconnection she most feared, since Ramona felt the need to distance herself from Jan's "helpful intrusions."

These interactive sequences are commonplace, and reworking this kind of troubled communication can comprise the bulk of the early work in therapy with what are termed "conflictual" couples. Many couple therapists have conceptualized these conflicts as resulting from projective identification processes (Catherall, 1992). In relational terms, the communication partners employ contains both a strategy of disconnection and a simultaneous attempt at connection, usually around old relational images. It is a fairly common way for couples to communicate in everyday life, particularly when one or both are experiencing grave discomforts (conscious or unconscious) with certain feeling states, and then with expressing, making known, such thoughts or feelings. The problem occurs when the *couple*, as a system, is unable to manage the difficult thoughts and feelings. The task of the couple's therapist is not just to help the agitated "provocateur" own his or her disavowed feelings, but also to build something between the couple—by helping the other understand, and have some empathy for, what is being projected onto him or her; or, absent any empathy, by encouraging him or her, at least, to respond to the other's distress and not dismiss it summarily as "That's *your* issue, and you need to work on it." Ultimately, the task is to identify and clarify the shared feelings, to differentiate their sources and causes, and to feel or empathize with them more accurately in oneself and one another.

All of us can probably recall numerous incidences, in our own intimate encounters, of times where we were agitated about something, unable to articulate it, and would try to "get" our partner to know what we were feeling. If our partner were unable to empathize with our agitation—giving a response such as, "That doesn't worry me, why are you so upset?"—then we were naturally left feeling alone and misunderstood. One could say person A should have done a better job of expressing what he or she was really feeling—"If you had said what you were feeling, then I could have responded better"—but in a couplehood, it is just as important that person B develop a capacity to feel or empathize with A's distress, in part, by B's awareness of his or her own feelings, as they are stimulated by A. In that way, each person is not left alone to puzzle it out and work on individual vulnerabilities but can join, as one member of a couple, in a mutual effort to be helpful to each other when faced with difficult feelings.

The times when Jan was worried about Ramona's productivity she fairly burst at the seams, more with anxiety about herself than for Ramona, fearful that her own essential strategies of disconnection would be overwhelmed. As Jan was opening up more in her individual therapy, particularly around the surgeries and her sexual fantasies, her fears of no longer being the "strong, accomplished one" could lead *her* to spiral downward into the dark underbelly of her "weak, needy" self and the accompanying self-loathing. If Jan could no longer work and produce—that is, make herself feel capable, strong and competent—then she would be worthless. No one could possibly want her then.

When a hint of this "weakness" appeared in either her or Ramona, Jan had to squash it. Week after week, when Jan would fuss about Ramona, I would gently but firmly steer Jan toward herself, suggesting that there was something that *she* was worried about in herself, and that I wanted to hear about it. Jan would scoff at both the suggestion that *she* was worried, and at my stated interest in her, attempting to dismiss the anxiety-provoking focus on herself. At this point, the reproaches had lost some of their punch. We had had enough contact to develop a shared, beginning sense that neither of us was going anywhere. And on Ramona's part, with some support, she was able to move, fairly quickly, out of a disconnected, counterblaming stance and gently, but persistently, ask Jan to talk about her own fears. Ramona then worked to respond to these fears in a manner that involved disclosing her own real concerns about not being productive, how bad it made her feel, and her own worries about the potential consequences of failing to get her writing done. Gradually, these interchanges moved them toward the ability to experience some mutual empathy, as each saw in the other what they were also struggling with in themselves, and went a long way toward building a much needed closeness, as they experienced being understood at the places where they felt most vulnerable.

THE RELATIONSHIP'S IMPACT ON THE THERAPIST

Watching this movement, and in some ways being a part of it, I felt something being jarred loose within me. In the presence of Jan and Ramona sharing authentically what were previously hidden feelings, and thereby letting go of some disconnecting ways of relating, I felt optimism for them and myself. I had been brought along, opened up to new possibilities. Little did I know that the chance to engage these "new possibilities" was coming at me, right down the pike. Needless to say, whatever is happening with the couple is not just confined to the dyadic relation. Depending on his or her valences, the therapist, as well, is able to receive and participate in the wellspring of feelings arising from old relational images. It is sometimes safest for the therapist to see the emotionality as being "just between the couple," a notion buttressed by the fact that that is where a lot of the work should be focused; helping the couple manage *their* interchanges.

As I felt a growing connection with Jan and Ramona, which was aided by my identification with some of their core dilemmas, as well as by their fairly consistent display of humor, warmth, and investment, I became more aware of my own feelings and reactions. I did not have to steel myself against them. Coincident with the work they were doing, I was becoming more able to reflect on myself and let previously quieted, difficult feelings emerge. The interactions we had around Jan "dismissing" my concern, and my being able to identify with her actual fear of *being dismissed*, as it was happening right there in the room with her, brought me into the mire.

In order to be empathic with Jan's anxiety, I first had to understand my own. Sometimes I would feel utterly cast aside by Jan. This feeling would evoke old, painful relational images for me, and in this hard place, I did not expect a good resolution. An anxiety would surge forward. In protective response came the desire to leave or retaliate—to dismiss Jan in reaction to her dismissing me—and, unfortunately, that would sometimes occur. This pushing away had the desired effect, however momentarily, leading to a disconnection between Jan and me, which effectively shut us down. Once this disconnection was achieved, a new unrest would develop: the rumblings of hurt and anger about the rupture. Shortly thereafter, a desire to reconnect would ensue. Often, it would take the form of Jan or Ramona calling me on what had just happened; they would engage me in a way that felt respectfully challenging. Most often, the action taken by Jan following the disconnection was done in the service of connection, in an attempt to understand me so that I would understand her better, as well as for Jan to understand herself more fully—through her effect on me.

Many interchanges occurred in which Jan felt angry and misunderstood by me, because I had pushed her too fast or too hard to talk about material (primarily her sexuality and the surgeries) she did not feel ready to address, and then failed to be there for her in any helpful manner when she felt so utterly exposed and vulnerable. Most of this trauma material was being worked on in her individual therapy, and it was just starting to peek out in the couple's sessions. How far to go with coaxing this material into the couple's work was sometimes only ascertained by her cries of "That's enough! Can't you see how hard this is?!!"—but, by that point, I had already crossed the line. We were in pretty rocky terrain. It was hard enough for her to navigate it solo; to let someone join her in that journey complicated it immensely. In this world of her sexual thoughts and desires, she not only struggled with her own self-loathing but with the images of tormentors and inept handholders. It was inevitable that I would become both to her.

Accordingly, many difficult and important sessions were spent trying to determine what she needed from Ramona and me to help her talk about her sexual life and the traumatic medical procedures. How to help her in this endeavor was not something to be defined in an easy "to-do" list. We all were left with that common experience in trauma work that talking about the trauma is itself retraumatizing. I knew when Jan was approaching her limit; she would fix me with that glare and make numerous comments about my ineptness and utter failure to understand how terrible talking about this felt for her. At my better times, I could hear what she was saying, stop myself, collect all the images I had of what I knew she had been through—the more detailed information was given to me, with her consent, by her individual therapist—and realize that *I* was distressed about her pain and wanted to get her through it quickly, at a pace she sensibly was not going to sustain. I knew that Jan felt unsafe; her anger and dismissal of me were the only ways she had of exerting control and stopping a process that was beginning to feel harrowing. At other times, I was less understanding. I became oppositional when Jan would angrily chastise me for, say, using the wrong word. Before I could close my mouth, out would come that same word again. I rebelled against having my hands tied, of having to say "just the right thing in just the right way." I would not do what she consciously wanted me to do now, but I would do what she wanted to do as a scared young child—get out from under the constraints of others.

Largely, I could accept and understand these communications: her angry dismissal of me in an effort to protect herself and my resistance to being constrained by her. I felt reassured that Jan and I had enough history with each other for us to repair the disconnections in either that session or in the weeks to come. But there were also times when Jan's dismissive anger felt different and put me back on my heels. At these times, I would become angry that my best intentions were not appreciated; I would think to myself, "I should hardly be expected to read her mind." Silently, I felt hurt and as inept as charged: "If only I had been paying better attention." And, deep down, I felt banished. If my anger about this came through (usually in some joke about Jan's criticalness), or I expressed my hurt by withdrawing, it did not go unnoticed. I knew instantly, almost viscerally, like a day of reckoning, that how I managed my response would be critical to the therapy. They were asking me to do with them what I was asking them to do with each other: to stay in connection when feeling hurt or angry; to not hide when afraid.

I would often get a call from Jan following such an interchange, or sometimes she would wait until the next session to bring it up. Directly and fairly accurately, she usually would comment about what she had seen in me (my discomfort, anger, or withdrawal) and how it had affected her. She would then invite me to share with her what had been going on with me during the session: why I felt the way I did. These were some of the more difficult conversations, but they were also the most alive. Sometimes I was able to respond better than others. When Jan's anxiety would line up with my own, it could be blinding. At those times, I would be unable to say what had been going on with me and would fumble some bland answer. But Jan and Ramona displayed a patience with me that I also gave to them. My self-challenge was to honestly acknowledge feeling inept and pushed away, and to figure out a way to talk about these feelings so that doing so would be useful for her. I would address the realities of how alone she sometimes felt and her need to protect herself. In this pained place, she would act in such a manner that paradoxically created what she was trying to prevent. She would chase me away and wind up alone. I was variably the inept mother—not able to foresee, understand, or help her in her pain; the hurtful surgeon—intruding upon her and causing her pain; or I was made to feel as the 7-year-old helpless child had felt— frozen, restrained, unable to move. It was how I worked with this latter relational image that was crucial to the therapy.

My reactions to Jan certainly captured, and then reflected, her experiences. But there was also something of me in there as well. I have my own history of feeling tragically inept at caretaking, and, as we all have, my own hurts around being left out or abandoned. When Jan would push me aside, it was not just my effort to pull out of my injured retreat, managing the relational images and shaking off their restraint, which was important for her to see. The task was not for me to silently struggle with and "master" alone what I was feeling. Rather, it was our combined effort—and how her empathy for me helped me to move into a different place—that could then lead Jan to an experience of increased self-empathy. There was a pressure in her questions to respond differently, to share some of my reactions, to think about my effect on her and her effect on me. It was a different interaction for both of us; one of wanting and connecting in these lonely, afraid places, rather than continuing to hide.

These moments capture the essence of what the Stone Center theorists describe as the process of mutuality:

> For the therapist, mutuality refers to a way of being in relationship, empathically attuned, emotionally responsive, authentically present and open to change. The therapist's growth in the relationship involves enhanced empathic possibilities, capacities to stay present with a range of difficult and complex feelings within herself and others, and greater freedom to stay in the process and bring more and more of herself into the relationship. (Surrey, 1997, p. 43)

Mutuality does not always happen in an even, graceful flow, and it is often the client's confrontation of the therapist's form of disconnecting that compels it forward. The client's equal need to know who we are, to have us participate in the relationship, to feel that he or she can understand us, even give to us, is often the root of mutuality's emergence. To allow clients to give of themselves (their empathy, their kindness) and to feel empowered in those capacities are essential experiences for their growth and the development of the therapy. It is important not to maintain a unilateral stance that therapy is all about the therapist knowing, understanding, and giving to the client.

In the beginning stages, it was hard helping Ramona articulate her concerns, hurts, and desires to Jan. Ramona is more elusive; she would drift away from herself by joining me in a contemplative, searching focus on Jan. As noted, I frequently experienced Ramona as my ally, and since this was a welcome support, I initially failed to question what meaning this alliance had for her, their relationship, or my relationship with Ramona, not to mention Jan. Of course, her attending to Jan in this manner was important in its own right: It was key to building a much needed foundation of intimacy and support, particularly around the trauma work. As a couple's therapist, though, there must be sensitivity to issues of balance in the sessions. We must pay attention to our alliance (liking one more than the other), our identifications (feeling more like one than the other), or just a simple accounting of how much "air time" each individual is getting. This does not mean merely trying to ensure that each person gets equal attention. It is not a question of equality; it is a matter of empathic attunement to each individual's needs, an assessment of the developmental stage of the therapy, and a discernment of where the appropriate focus needs to be.

A lot of the work in the beginning and middle phases of therapy had been on Jan. Particularly as the therapy moved in and out of the trauma material, Ramona and I served as significant witnesses (see Johnson, 1998). Ramona gained much from this role. Jan's work and Ramona's supportive involvement had certainly deepened their relationship, which benefited them both. Nonetheless, I would sometimes find myself at the end of the session distinctly feeling that we had learned a lot about Jan, but not much about Ramona—except for her proclivity to attend to Jan and to be "helpful" to me. It is not that she refused to participate but that she would get her attention primarily *through* Jan, almost vicariously. When Ramona would bring up something special, particular to her, none of us would take off and run with it in a sustained way. There did not seem to be the same urgency. She did not seem to need much. But, lingering in the back of my mind, as I had learned in working with their difficult conflict processes, was Ramona's ability to empathize with Jan's fear of being unwanted. Ramona did not have Jan's feeling that she was "disgusting and loathsome," but from her own earlier experiences, she was afraid of going unnoticed and feeling inconsequential; of others "turning their heads away." It was enacted in the therapy. It came to us. She would bring up something special to her, and I, essentially, "turned my head."

There was Ramona's contribution to this—her reticence to insert herself—as well as Jan's involvement in not looking, being sometimes too involved in her own work or anxiety to notice Ramona. Then there was my neglect. It is with a certain amount of guilt that I write about those patients who please me by their accommodation, how they gratify me by not asking for much. Ramona is one of them. This is one of my central adaptations—making myself scarce. It is how I learned to move through the world, and I am unfortunately still most comfortable with it in others and myself. As was the case with Jan, in my effort to better know Ramona in the areas that were difficult for her, I had to be more known and willing to struggle in the identical areas of difficulty for me. I have had to work much harder, pursue her more, in order to get in and connect up with her vulnerable places. Part of that is her doing; she does not ask for much and stays back easily. But part of that, I know, is my doing. Going after a patient challenges me, because I have to feel *my* needs first. I have to *want* to reach that client and to put my desire into action. Wanting others and laying that wanting out there is thorny for me. It is also Ramona's primary challenge—to go after others. I knew that if I was to help her with this area, I would have to grow as well. I would have to want her more openly, and in order to become more open, I would have to trust her. If I did not go after her, this relational reticence was not going to change—for her or for me.

Again, they pressed this hesitancy of mine with me, as I pressed it with Ramona—in a humorous, but very direct way: around the seating arrangement in the office. Traditionally, I sit in a chair opposite the couch, where they sit. Usually, Jan sits in the corner of the couch, directly across from me, and Ramona sits at the other end of the couch, kitty-corner from me. One day they arrived, having discussed over the week that it would now be Ramona's turn to sit opposite me, which she did (and still does). This change led to several fruitful discussions about Ramona's need to be more attended to; about how it was difficult for her, when sitting in the other position, to claim her time on center stage. She had been so aware of what transpired between Jan and me, and found herself reacting as the outsider, on the periphery. Being in this new "spot," which many couples describe as the "hot seat," allowed her to look at either Jan or me and not have to consider the panorama. I felt complicit and embarrassed, aware that I had "let this happen," that something as physical and dramatic as changing seats had to occur to *them* for me to awaken. I did not feel that I had to push through any anxiety to meet her, as I do at times with Jan. Instead, I felt sadness, almost a grief, which engulfed me as I became more aware of her aloneness and my own. With increasing clarity, I began to see and feel Ramona's history of being left alone, and my contribution to her feeling alone, by my need to avoid those feelings in myself. Though sad, I also felt opened up and relieved, and I wanted to hear more about these times in her life. I did not disclose any particulars about my own experiences with aloneness. Ramona responded to my affect with what has always been her trademark: firm, exquisite sensitivity. She welcomed me in, to join her in these sad places. Again, as in these moments of mutuality with Jan, there was a feeling that Ramona and I were meeting in, and responding to, these protected and lonely places in each other. There was an opening, a softening, which led to an increase in mutual empathy, as well as self-empathy.

Ramona took to this new seating arrangement, and Jan has largely supported the move, remarking that one of the benefits of the couple's therapy, for her, has been to hear more about what is going on with Ramona, to be let into her life. Ramona can be a woman of few words and typically does not disclose much, unless pressed. She began to talk about herself more openly and consistently, in a way that made me much more aware of her. She complained more vigorously about Jan's lapses into self-absorption, and how sad and left out she felt at times. But she readily looked at her struggles with making herself visible. Incidents that occurred throughout the week were recounted. We discussed events they had attended or evenings spent together when Ramona felt the focus had been on Jan and her needs. In the sessions, with some encouragement, Jan was able to shift and join in, focusing on Ramona, nudging and inviting her to come forward, expressing clear interest: "I am here. Just come." Having done a lot of this work on the receiving end with Ramona, Jan was now better positioned to be on the giving end. She was increasingly able to respond empathically to Ramona's stated needs for more recognition and attention.

MOVING DEEPER INTO CONNECTION

About 3 years into the therapy, the attempts to vanquish unwanted feelings by active warring and prolonged and rigid forms of disengagement had largely ceased. Jan and Ramona had enough new experiences with each other to counter the old relational images and fortify us to move deeper. Additionally, a pattern of relational awareness (see Jordan, 1995) had been cultivated, wherein we were each better able to clarify what we felt, to know better what the other was feeling, and to have greater appreciation for our impact on each other. "Good conflict" or "engaged conflict" (Pinsof, 1995) was emerging. Jan and Ramona began to bring themselves forward in a stronger way. They no longer spent the sessions complaining primarily about the other. Rather, they were able to move into spaces within themselves, recognize their own longings and unmet needs, as well as the other's, and begin to speak from there. This enhanced ability to relate more fully and authentically was also due to ongoing work in their individual therapies. The couple's work would never have achieved this level without the benefit of their individual work. A wonderful synergy between the individual and couple's work had brought us this far.

A connection had solidified in which the natural quest for growth could occur: There was a mutual investment and energy in representing themselves more fully, which included the opportunities for both getting more as well as giving more. This led, fairly naturally, into an enlarged discussion of their sexual relationship. Ramona began asking for more responsiveness to her sexual needs, and Jan began a fuller description of her difficulties in the sexual realm. Jan was clear that having sex made her feel awful. Due to the trauma of the surgeries, her sexual life was encapsulated in trauma-ridden fantasies, resulting in profound shame. For Jan, having sex was not making love, and it felt next to impossible to engage in sexual contact with Ramona. They were physical and increasingly affectionate, but did not engage in any genital contact, or prolonged kissing or touching that might lead to a state of arousal.

Feeling an increased capacity to move forward with their intimate needs, including a desire to be responsive to the other, Jan and Ramona collaborated in pushing the sexual relationship forward as an area for discussion in the couple's session, despite mounting anxiety. This was the final tug on the lid of Pandora's box, and we circled back to the beginning anxieties: for Jan, the incredible humiliation and fear she experienced in going to the remembered trauma and the accompanying self-loathing; for Ramona, the fear and despair that was felt around longings for connection; and for me, the fear and distress associated with feeling abandoned and unable to connect. We revisited the basic fear for all of us: The more one wants and needs, the more threatened one feels. These were some of the more difficult, though inspiring, times for me, as we struggled to remain present to each other and forge a connection in such profound places of shame and despair. In the throes of terror and shame, Jan would question, "Is going through this, is talking about this, really going to help?" To see her curled up, pounding her head, made me both doubt the helpfulness of the process and feel partially the cause of her pain. I would feel like one of her earlier professional tormentors. Finding a way to be with her and Ramona at these times presented the same challenges as before, but more insistently, as Jan attended to the trauma material more directly. She needed to feel that I could be with her in a stronger, clearer way. Sometimes this has involved my sitting next to her on the couch, to provide a safety net at these crucial moments. She needed me to keep her from going into, what she terms, "free fall"; to provide a platform to catch her spiral downward. My physical presence—holding her hand or putting an arm around her shoulder—would let her know I was there, at those times when words could not reach her.

I still had not been able to gauge consistently what she wanted from me, and, as before, would find out that I had over- or undershot the mark after the fact. Either I was too far away (distant, removed) or too close (insistent) in a hurtful way. These "missteps" have given us many fruitful opportunities: to explore the relational ruptures she experienced around the trauma and address those ruptures in a reparative relational manner, providing a sorely missed empathy for the pain and fear she experienced; and the opportunity for her to now have control over her emotional needs with others. Informed by much practice, we can now negotiate this territory and the disconnections that develop much better. For example, Jan has begun to catch her desire to flee, by chasing others away, commenting, "I know what I'm doing now. I'm just trying to find anything I can to be mad at you or Ramona about!" And I have become more aware of my feelings of being dismissed or inept and what they are about, and of the continued need to grapple with them in a way other than retreating. To this aim, I often call to mind the story I read about the composer Stravinsky:

> He had written a new piece with a difficult violin passage. After it had been in rehearsal for several weeks, the solo violinist came to Stravinsky and said he was sorry, he had tried his best, the passage was too difficult; no violinist could play it. Stravinsky said, "I understand that. What I am after is the sound of someone *trying* to play it." (Powers, 1984, p. 54, in Mitchell, 1988, p. 293)

The vignette reminds me of a central aspect of therapeutic endeavor: that it is rare and often unnecessary to reach an exact understanding of one's client, but it is critical to be engaged in the process of trying.

As we work with Jan's trauma material, weaving it in and out of the sessions to integrate it, Ramona has not been lost. She remains consistently attentive to Jan, and we work on altering her tendency to submerge herself in Jan's work. Generally, Ramona now comes into the session more forcefully, wanting to talk about herself, about something she wants and needs. She is less afraid to be noticed or to express her desires, and she demonstrates this new forthrightness in numerous ways. In her professional life, she committed to a big writing project; in her relationship with Jan, she continues to long openly for increased attention to her needs; and with me, she persists in getting the needed attention. With

Ramona, the continued challenge has been to keep tabs on my "hands off" posture, and to keep her from her own free fall, not landing with a thud as Jan would, but quietly drifting away. Helping her requires me to be vigilant toward my own counterdependent stance. I need to remind myself that, as possibilities increase for her to get more, it is imperative for me to stay in there with her longings, and to depotentiate both of our allegiances to that old saw: Aspiring for closeness means risking disappointment.

We continue in the therapy, and the relationships feel solid. We have used many active water metaphors in our work ("Jump in!" "Dive off," "Don't keep your head down, look up and notice me on the pier," and "I'll move over into another lap lane and make room for you, if you would just get in!"). To describe the therapy relationship as feeling weathered seems fitting. We have been through drizzle, steady rains, squalls, skies opening to the warmth of the sun, more storms. We are past the question of "Is it worth it, is there something to be gained?" We have all benefited from the therapy, and want more. Recently, Jan and Ramona have begun to describe stories of coming together in a different way. They have found more of the "we" in the relationship, and it feels to them less like "she and I." They engage in more collaboration, whether in discussing a vacation, planning financially for retirement (which they had never done jointly, just thought about individually), or making a major purchase together. There is a different quality to the relationship. They used to feel that the only way to be in relationship was by keeping aspects of themselves out.

We now know better.

REFERENCES

Bergman, S., & Surrey, J. (1992). The woman–man relationship: Impasses and possibilities. *Work in Progress, No. 55*. Wellesley, MA: Stone Center Working Paper Series.

Catherall, D. (1992). Working with projective identification in couples. *Family Process, 31*, 355–367.

Gottman, J., & Silver, N. (2000). *The seven principles for making marriage work*. New York: Three Rivers Press.

Herman, J. (1992). *Trauma and recovery*. New York: Basic Books.

Johnson, S. (1996). *The practice of emotionally focused therapy: Creating connection*. New York: Brunner/Mazel.

Johnson, S. (1998). Creating healing relationships for couples dealing with trauma: The use of emotionally focused marital therapy. *Journal of Marital and Family Therapy, 24*(1), 25–40.

Jordan, J. (1995). Relational awareness: Transforming disconnection. *Work in Progress, No. 76*. Wellesley, MA: Stone Center Working Paper Series.

Miller, A. (1981). *The drama of the gifted child*. New York: Basic Books.

Miller, J. B. (1999). Therapist's authenticity. *Work in Progress, No. 82*. Wellesley, MA: Stone Center Working Paper Series.

Miller, J. B., & Stiver, I. P. (1997). *The healing connection: How women form relationships in therapy and in life*. Boston: Beacon Press.

Mitchell, S. (1988). *Relational concepts in psychoanalysis: An integration*. Cambridge, MA: Harvard University Press.

Pinsof, W. (1995). *Integrative problem-centered therapy: A synthesis of family, individual and biological therapies*. New York: Basic Books.

Pinsof, W. (2000). *Transforming conflict and building love*. Postgraduate Education Programs, The Family Institute at Northwestern University, Evanston, IL.

Real, T. (2002). *How can I get through to you: Reconnecting men and women*. New York: Scribner.

Schnarch, D. (1997). *Passionate marriage*. New York: Norton.

Surrey, J. (1997). What do you mean by mutuality in therapy? In J. V. Jordan (Ed.), *Women's growth in diversity: More writings from the Stone Center* (pp. 42–46). New York: Guilford Press.

8

Moving toward "We"
Promise and Peril

KAREN SKERRETT

Mick and Elise are a midlife, affluent, professional couple who have been married for 14 years. Both have achieved considerable prominence in their respective fields. They have two children together, a son age 12 and a daughter age 9. Mick, at 47, had been married previously for 12 years and has a college-age daughter and son. He maintains a "friendly," collaborative relationship with his former wife, despite chronic dissatisfaction with her style of parenting their children. At 51, this is Elise's first marriage. She describes a good relationship with Mick's former wife and feels closely connected to both stepchildren. Elise initially called requesting couple counseling, saying that Mick was threatening to move out unless things changed, and she had "no idea" where to start or what to do.

The attractive couple that appeared in my office shortly thereafter immediately drew me to their contrasting styles. Mick was colorfully dressed, warm, engaging (albeit anxious), and funny. Elise was reserved, serious, tightly controlled, fastidiously and darkly dressed, giving her an aura of severity. As we began the getting-acquainted process, their contrasting energies intensified: chaos/calm, loose/rigid, aggressive/controlled. As I struggled to find my own point of balance in this system, Mick seemed very anxious about "getting" (approval, air time, soothing),

128

whereas Elise seemed lost yet hypervigilant in trying to assess what Mick and I might want from her. As I listened to their unfolding story, filled with loss, great pain, isolation, and longing, I felt myself responding at a deep level to this pair.

PRESENTING CONCERNS

Mick's complaints dominated the room. He spoke of feeling depressed and either chronically angry or having panic attacks. He felt at the end of his ability to tolerate a marriage "without warmth or affection." Although both were professionally successful, he continued, their personal life was a "vacuum." They worked constantly, "ministered" to their children, and had "no relationship." He claimed having tried "everything" to please Elise over the years. Most recently, he was in a new phase of "withdrawal" to try to focus on himself, but he was finding that just as painful as the earlier attempts to get Elise to meet his needs. Elise did not want the marriage to fail but usually felt "overwhelmed" by Mick's neediness. She thoroughly enjoyed her work and viewed Mick as frequently a "great father." She also carefully volunteered that she thought an antianxiety medication would help Mick, especially in coping with what she saw as unrealistic expectations of himself, her, and the marriage, compounded by an "out-of-proportion" feeling of failure.

Neither had had prior therapy, with the exception of several family sessions 5 years earlier, triggered by the depression of Mick's oldest son. Despite their contrasting styles of expression and containment, the pain and despair in the room was palpable. They alternated between expressing feelings of their "absolute need for help" and their hopelessness that they might be "beyond repair."

Both Mick and Elise responded favorably to my reformulation of their complaints as exactly what happens when couples suffer from chronic disconnection (Miller & Stiver, 1997). After a brief analysis of their genogram, they could see how they were, in fact, embedded within layers of disconnection: Mick from his father and brother; Elise from her mother, father, and stepfather; both from their children and their friends; and most essential of all—from themselves.

Both resonated to the language of connection/disconnection and admitted that they clearly lacked a sense of well-being, felt paralyzed vis-à-vis one another in the relationship, and were chronically unsure about what they and the other wanted and/or needed. Neither felt very worthy in the eyes of the other, and although Mick claimed a longing to feel more connected with Elise, it was obvious that both were terrified by the prospects.

From the very beginning, I introduced and then continued to develop the notion of the relationship as a third entity: I, you, and the relationship (Shem & Surrey, 1998). As is common for most couples, in my experience, Mick and Elise came to therapy with a very independent view of their marriage, approaching issues from the perspective of their individual (though seldom articulated) wants and needs. They were unaware that, for better or worse, every behavioral choice they made had consequences for the relationship. Thus, I identified myself in the role of guardian of the relationship. In that role I would use every opportunity to help them become more conscious of their individual responses and the implications of those responses for the immediate and long-term vitality of the relationship. Also, I told them I would strive to take responsibility for my own reactions and to share them in ways intended to clarify and keep the collaborative process of therapy moving forward. Initially, I spent a fair amount of time clarifying the "we" in reference at any given time; was this the "we" of the couple twosome or the "we" of the three-way collaborative effort? For example, assigning weekly homework to spend 30 minutes of uninterrupted time together nourished the "we" of the couple twosome; bringing into sessions their leftover questions or reactions from the previous week facilitated the process of teamwork between the three of us. The idea of the "we" became a powerful ally in change, particularly early in our work when reactivity was especially high. Asking them to pause and reflect on the impact an immediate, strong reaction might have, not just on the other but for the relationship, developed their capacity for observation and fostered the safety that helped deescalate tensions. Over time, we regularly referenced the state of the "we," asking, for example, "How is this new 'we'?" and "What might be done to nurture this changing "we'?" (Shem & Surrey, 1998).

CORE FACILITATIVE PROCESSES

My work with Mick and Elise reflects my understanding that the processes of relational movement (essentially connection/disconnection/deeper connection) drive change in the context of couple therapy (Miller, 2001; Skerrett, 1996, 2003). I visualize this movement and the related facilitation processes as a spiral, in which the elements evolve in a fluid, interdependent way. Many changes can happen simultaneously to deepen levels of mutual authenticity and connectedness to self and other. The facilitative processes are (1) the creation of safety, (2) facilitating authenticity and shared vulnerability, (3) increasing ownership of feelings and recognition of feelings in others, and (4) reworking relational images to connect across difference.

The Creation of Safety

Most couples begin therapy feeling some degree of frustration, disappointment, and blame toward self and other and are frightened to risk sharing their real experience of the relationship. I immediately try to create a climate conducive to identifying and speaking genuine feelings. When done at a pace that is respectful of each person's need for protection, a climate of safety is increasingly created. Blame is routinely redirected toward developmental and cultural factors.

Facilitating Authenticity and Shared Vulnerability

I encourage authenticity and shared vulnerability by striving to bring myself into the room as clearly and authentically as possible from the outset. I also challenge the culturally prescribed image of intimacy (Real, 1997) as a perpetual state to be achieved and maintained, instead defining intimacy for the couple as a momentary experience of shared empathy, authenticity, and deepened connection (Miller & Stiver, 1997). As mutual honesty increases, constraining images, ideas, and illusions are identified. Often, disappointments intensify as partners begin to recognize they cannot "make" the other person change. Simultaneously, the capacity for tolerating individual and relational truths (self and other) and repairing mutual injury grows as each partner brings greater authenticity into the relationship. Intrinsic to this development is ownership.

Increasing Ownership of Feelings and the Capacity to Recognize the Feelings of Others

When couples are distressed and disconnected, they often feel confused about which feelings belong to whom. Much of the work of the therapy involves helping each partner clarify and "own" his or her feelings and learn to recognize and empathize with the feelings of the partner. Gaining this sense of ownership also involves helping the partners find new ways to understand and then honor an altered view of self and other.

Reworking Relational Images and Connecting across Difference

This is at the heart of what moves the therapy: attempting to articulate the relational images that have given meaning to, and structured, each individual's world and relationships. I assist couples to identify old images and build more resilient ones (Jordan, 1992). As this process unfolds, each person develops an increasing capacity for personal expansiveness and a greater ability to connect across differences.

THE CREATION OF SAFETY

The first and most essential element needed to begin the healing process for this profoundly isolated couple was the creation of safety. Unless and until they could experience our three-way relationship as a place of safety, where their vulnerabilities would be protected, as opposed to exploited, they would not begin to reestablish the mutual sense of good will so essential to any risk taking.

One of the central ways I attended to this task was by weaving back and forth between a focus on immediate concerns (about self and other) and attempting to embed those concerns within the broader context of their lives and the relational images that have evolved. Proceeding in this way helped mitigate the tendency toward fault finding and contextualized the pain in such a way that they could begin to feel less "crazy," isolated, and hopeless (Skerrett, 1996, 1997, 2003). For example, it was very helpful to provide the information that many couples struggle with the degree of closeness/distance needed by each, and that these needs are highly influenced by experiences in each person's family of origin and "normally" shift over time and with a couple's experiences with one another. This alternative perspective gave them a new way to think about themselves and each other, other than in terms of mutual criticism and blame.

To begin the process of helping the partners redirect this tendency toward individualized and isolated blame, we identified the developmental and cultural factors that shaped and constrained their perspectives (Madsen, 1999). For example, they were beginning (particularly Mick) to respond to the shifting "developmental imperative" (Nemiroff & Colarusso, 1990)—awareness of a shorter time left to live and a related reexamination of how that time might be spent. Mick, as the oldest son of a first-generation blue-collar Irish family, could never do anything right in the eyes of his father. Mick's professional status as an adult threatened his father and was dismissed as "not counting for much." Several birth defects—small cleft lip, obvious leg and hip deformities, and a serious lisp—contributed to Mick's belief that he was deserving of the physical beatings he had withstood throughout his childhood. The mother, whom he adored, died suddenly when Mick was 16. For Elise, the third daughter of a wealthy, prominent East Coast "blue-blood" family, failure was not a word in the household vocabulary, and little was given but much was expected. All of her siblings were highly successful professionals; with each remarriage, her mother has "moved up the ladder of affluence." However, neither Elise's childhood nor current-day accomplishments are acknowledged—only imperfections. I began to understand Elise's protective shell once she started offering short, clipped stories of her mother commenting on her "ugly outfit" or "stupid vacation plan" or her father criticizing her hair style or choice of dinner menu.

Both Mick and Elise had embodied this country's dictate of success at all costs. Both held many earned and unearned privileges. By virtue of her birth into a wealthy, Caucasian professional family of "old-money" stature, Elise personified a history of unearned privilege. Mick's history, as the son of Caucasian lower-middle-class working parents, was less privileged than Elise's, despite the culturally conferred advantage of race and gender. Both Mick and Elise held prestigious jobs that brought multiple earned privileges. Nevertheless, they were currently as much hostages to their lifestyle as are people with considerably fewer resources. Mick, in particular, talked about his occasional spending "binges" as attempts to convince himself that he was "having fun." One weekday, he impulsively left his office and bought several thousands of dollars worth of electronics so that he could "fantasize about someday really using them." More often, he just felt deprived and generally came home so exhausted that he had no energy to enjoy what he did have.

At the point when they entered therapy, Mick was expressing considerably more disillusionment with their mutual workaholism, finding it no balm to the feelings of failure and increasing dissonance with the changing needs of midlife. Elise initially expressed greater contentment with her work–home balance, but also had a considerable investment in appearing able to "do it all." They understood how the general feeling of being "out of control" of their lifestyle contributed to the tendency of both to hold the other accountable for their dissatisfaction and to experience a lack of safety with one another. They tended to approach this issue of mutual overwork, as most other issues, in an "all-or-nothing" fashion: for example, "Either I cut my hours to part time or tell the partners I want out." Both spouses had great difficulty formulating a compromise position to their either/or mindset. Likewise, both held relational images of isolation and emotional deprivation. Believing that there was no one outside themselves who could be counted on, each subscribed to strong individualistic rather than interdependent strategies. Thus it was a common experience in our sessions for each to contribute a "solution" to whatever problem was on the table. However, lacking the relational imagery to support collaboration and the tools to bring it about, they would end up feeling disconnected and locked in a futile dynamic where nothing was ever really resolved. Early in our work, we jointly developed a plan for Mick to cut back his schedule one half day per week and for Elise to lend verbal support and be available for couple outings. Before Mick enacted this plan, we identified the possible ways in which he might let himself down and positioned our work as a resource to help him fulfill his commitment to both himself and the relationship. We talked about the ways Elise could support him in making this lifestyle change. Being able to commit to this small change felt very relieving to both Mick and Elise and not only strengthened our alliance but began to give them a renewed sense of control over the course and quality of their life together.

In a related fashion, we examined their gender roles and the ways in which their expectations of self and other contributed to feeling stuck, unsafe, and out of balance. Although exhibiting a quality of gender reversal on one level ("She wears the pants—I'm the needy one"), their roles in the relationship clearly reflected the way in which our culture trains boys/ men not to tolerate stress in themselves and for girls/women to protect others from feeling stress. Elise's family history reinforced this cultural dictate to protect men. Her mother modeled a demeanor of stony silence in response to Elise's father's flagrant infidelities and unethical professional conduct. Although out-of-control men made Elise feel very frightened, her typical reserved and stoic stance mirrored her mother's and served the dual purpose of protecting her own anxiety as well as Mick's. Having grown up with a violent father, Mick felt very anxious around any sign of disapproval or anger. Thus, if Elise did not get in touch with her frustration/anger or bring it into the relationship, then neither would Mick, and the partnership was felt to be safer by both.

Often, I found myself wondering what Elise must be feeling or thinking, but if I gave her too much attention, she grew even more uncomfortable. It was as if they had an unspoken agreement that the relationship could only manage so much affect, and Mick was the designated "holder." Clearly, both were very organized around managing Mick's anxiety level. No matter what the issue under discussion, he was the more reactive, and at those times Elise would become even more silent. Both acted as if the most important point was for Mick to get some relief. Although I agreed with Elise that medication would be a benefit to Mick, reducing his overall level of agitation, sleeplessness, and ruminations, it was more essential that he be allowed to let me bear his distress with him. I believed that the governing relational image shared by all three of us was that there is no one, outside of self, who can be counted on to help get needs met. I strongly identified with the resulting loneliness, isolation, and desperation and was fortunate to have had positive experiences of allowing myself to be helped by others. I wanted to begin to provide such an alternative emotional experience for them and to demonstrate that shared pain can decrease isolation, deepen connection, and promote healing. Furthermore, for Elise I wanted to facilitate a different understanding of the origins and meaning of Mick's pain, through her witnessing of my work with him.

Six months into the treatment, Mick did accept a referral for a medication consult and not only experienced symptom relief but a shift in Elise's capacity to relate to him. With her husband less worried about his ability to function, Elise began to expose more of herself and her concerns to him, and she was more willing to agree to some of Mick's requests for attention. However, Mick's relationship with medication has been problematic throughout the majority of treatment. He struggles periodically with intensified feelings of being a "crazy failure" and precipitously stops taking his medication. He also will cut or drop doses when angry with Elise because he knows it will make her very frustrated. I felt empathic with Mick's very real distress, and at the same time, I tried to help both of them feel safer by demonstrating my belief that Mick could manage his anxiety more effectively by taking responsibility for his medication and stop making medication management a relationship issue.

Since both partners initially tended to approach things intellectually, early psychoeducation about gender roles—the ways in which each gender is differentially socialized in this culture as well as information about the influence of early family models—also provided a new perspective that reduced blame, increased feelings of safety, and helped them think about alternative ways of responding to one another.

We used the language of connection/disconnection in relation to Mick's anxiety and reactivity, as it was very obvious that the effect of his heightened affect had a distancing effect, usually for Elise and frequently for me. Particularly at those times when I was aware of working hard to provide containment and soothing and he still felt overwhelmed, I disconnected into fantasies of telling him to "just knock it off!" I more fully identified with Elise's response to his neediness—retreating into silence and disconnection. Experiencing a client regularly and loudly agitate and demand to have his needs met raised my own anxiety. Clearly what Mick wanted the most—attention and emotional soothing—resulted in Elise's and, less often, my own withdrawal into disconnection, which then further heightened his anxiety (Jordan, 1995). Routinely pointing out the sequence, sharing my reactions, and encouraging Elise to share hers seemed to shift things, but often too slowly to suit me. Another of my own strategies of disconnection was impatience: If someone did not move along/ take my suggestion at the pace I thought he or she should (i.e., met my needs), I became irritated and disconnected. Similar to both Mick and Elise, this helped protect me from the vulnerable feelings of not having been appreciated—especially given how hard I tried.

One of Elise's early and related strategies of disconnection was one that Mick referred to as "pulling rank." During a session her pager would go off, and no matter what was happening in the room, she would stand, walk over to me, and ask to use my telephone. The first time it happened, I noted Mick's eye rolling and his comment to her, "Why don't you just use your cell phone out in the hall." The next time it happened, she was on the phone for several minutes, and Mick began complaining to me about how she "loves to control everything and could certainly turn off her pager during sessions" just as he did. I took a calculated risk and encouraged him to share his comment with Elise. Despite considerable reluctance, he shared a modified version of his feelings with Elise. She responded first (somewhat defensively) that she did not think of using her cell phone and never thought twice about most of what she did. I shared an awareness of my own discomfort in the room and jokingly offered to answer the call for her. I said I would prefer my more familiar role of being in charge. I shared that my desire to direct, take charge/take over, protected me from my own frustration and uncertainties over how to be helpful, and that I knew the impact of those responses was often distancing. The comment seemed to defuse the blame-saturated tension. Later, each offered the understanding that Elise's phone response was similar to Mick's reactivity. Both had the effect of distancing the other, and both were employed when Mick and Elise felt they had no other recourse to getting what they needed. I felt genuine empathy for both strategies, tried to model patience, and shared that when they felt safe enough, they would be ready to do something differently. After several months, Elise stopped bringing her pager to sessions and Mick began taking his medication more regularly.

MODELING: AUTHENTICITY/INTIMACY, SHARED VULNERABILITY

Both Mick and Elise were accomplished "performers"; that is, they tended to enact the role they thought was required rather than be themselves. Although I felt genuine respect for their achievements, I believed it essential to help them recognize the cost to their capacities for intimacy of their overreliance on their ability to perform. As a longstanding expert in overrelying on performance myself, I knew this focus would involve a mutual endeavor of the highest order. Mick, in particular, felt he needed to earn (i.e., perform for) whatever caretaking he received. This pattern was best symbolized early in our relationship through a coffee ritual. Typically, each came to sessions separately from different directions, and Mick usually passed a Starbucks on route. As he began to feel more connected to me and our work, he developed the habit of bringing in three cups of coffee. At first, I simply thanked him, then said it was not always necessary for him to treat me, tried humor ("You're my last appointment of the night—you don't really expect me to be awake and alert, do you?" etc.).

Then one week I brought in three cups of coffee. Both were surprised at first, then humored, then touched that I would reciprocate the gesture. That moment triggered an important dialogue in which Mick shared that he always felt he had to go "above and beyond" for people but that "enough was never enough"; he even ventured a beginning recognition of how burdening this felt to him. Elise volunteered that she often felt overwhelmed by Mick's unsolicited generosity because she felt, in part, that it was more about *him* than really for her. She experienced an undercurrent of demand, sensing that much was expected of her, but she never felt quite sure what exactly that was. She was further able to recognize how familiar that feeling of demand for who-knew-what was ("That was the story of my life growing up") and knew how very much she wanted to disconnect from it. Mick could begin to see that Elise's feelings explained why he felt chronically disappointed in her reactions. "I keep trying and trying, and I think I really do great stuff that she never appreciates." Understanding the link to her past—what was being triggered in the moment for her—helped him realize that she was not withholding from him, she was "trying to get away from the bad feelings inside." They could also begin to understand that it was this level of sharing—the truth-telling risk of expressing authentic feelings, as opposed to what each imagined was "required"—that characterized genuine connectedness: an intimate moment.

Another example of a critical juncture that facilitated considerable movement occurred 8 months into our work. Mick was still feeling a fair amount of anxiety, high stress at work and "deprived" and "unappreciated" at home. We began by talking about an incident that had happened that week at work, in which he felt criticized and misunderstood by one of his partners, and it had almost resulted in his "bungling a case." Mick's agitation increased as he described trying to talk to Elise about what had happened and getting her "businesslike I-don't-have-time-for-you-now shit." The more he talked, the more overwrought he became, and the more silent and frightened Elise looked. At one point, he jumped to his feet, saying he could not stay in a room or a marriage with someone so "cold and unresponsive." His desperation touched me deeply and resonated with my own history. I felt strongly that Mick's desperation needed to be seen and acknowledged with empathy and that it was critical for the movement of the therapy that he not leave the room. I stood with him, reached out to touch his arm and said that I felt something very important was happening and that we both needed him to try and stay with us to understand what that was. It took several attempts on my part for him to agree to sit back down, but as soon as he did, he dissolved into tears. I said that I knew how painfully frustrating it felt to try and try so hard to do well and then to not have those efforts recognized. He began to talk about how his father "never, ever once" gave him any credit for anything, and how he could not stop himself from trying to get his approval. Then he began to talk about how his mother was the only one who, he felt, knew and appreciated him, and he described with great poignancy how she would cradle him in her arms after one of the verbal lashings by his father, saying, "You're my wonderful Micky, you are so good and kind." He broke into sobs as he spoke about how desperately he missed her, how unfair it was to have lost her so young. I had felt exactly as Mick described his experience, having lost my own mother when I was a young adolescent. I had shared this part of my history during earlier sessions. Now I was deeply moved by Mick's pain and also sensed how moved he was to witness the effect his pain had on me. It felt intrusive and unnecessary to reference my history at this point and much more important that Mick stay with his experience. Elise was very quiet, but I knew that my vulnerability and willingness to expose it had had a profound impact on her. I sensed that Elise was resonating to our work out of her own history of loss, and I felt a mix of wonder and respect coming from her in response to my ability to demonstrate such empathy to Mick as well as to the ways in which Mick allowed himself to be comforted. I was hopeful that she would feel, perhaps, that I could also recognize the longings and vulnerabilities within her and respond compassionately. I felt strongly connected to both of them and took away a conviction that this work had moved both their relationship as well as the alliance between the three of us.

Several weeks after that session, the tenor of our work subtly changed. Mick began to recognize the feelings of desperation that would well up in him, what triggered them, and to what degree the feelings were embedded within the present or the past. He also tried to bring forth the feelings to Elise a bit earlier in the process of escalation and give her more time to respond. Because she better understood the meaning of his pain, she felt less "assaulted and personally responsible" and could feel more empathy and patience with his reactions. She also slowly began to share the briefest vignettes of the interactions with her own critical mother and how burdensome those experiences still felt. Mick typically saw Elise as invulnerable, highly competent, in perfect control, and disinterested in anyone else's feelings. To listen to her tentatively volunteer more about how she felt she could never please her mother, despite all her accomplishments, Mick was able to begin to understand that she was fearful of failing him and of being as criticized and diminished as she was by her mother. This revelation further expanded our growing climate of mutual empathy, as I too felt touched by their willingness to change and felt more deeply connected to each of them.

As they both began to feel more "real" to me, I found myself periodically aggravated and/or frustrated by our mutual retreats into disconnection. The retreats seemed most often triggered by their experience of disappointment or failure to meet one another's needs. Tolerance for disappointment was still quite low, so one or the other's unavailability or a harsh word between sessions might send each into a disconnect that would last until they walked into the next session. Sometimes, the retreat into the "superperformer" replication and reenactment (Miller & Stiver, 1997) would go on for weeks. I recognized my own expectations of perfection (as if it were possible to maintain perfect connection!), my own limits around staying fully engaged, and struggled to monitor my tendency to disconnect in the face of frustration and disappointment. I practiced self-empathy, telling myself it was OK if staying fully engaged was not possible. I tried, whenever I could, to bring my feelings into the room. I was not always clear on what enabled me to talk about my own strategies of disconnection at a particular time—perhaps a greater sense of openness to myself and more permission granting to be an imperfect therapist with two clients who preferred perfection. The following exchange was typical of this relational paradox:

KAREN: (*sounding bored, semi-frustrated, and irritated*) I'm wondering what might be happening now? We were talking about the argument you had on Sunday, and I felt we were gaining some understanding of how you each were feeling. Now I'm starting to feel distracted by what sounds like your complaints about what the other isn't doing. I'm having trouble listening.

MICK: Well, I'm just trying to get her to understand what it's like when she ignores what I'm saying and keeps doing what she's doing, like I'm not in the room.

ELISE: (*interrupting*) And I've told you over and over that I'm not ignoring you, I just don't know what it is you want.

KAREN: Let's all stop a minute and try to look at the sequence here . . . We were making headway in terms of sharing and listening to how hurt you each felt, and I was right there with you. Then something shifted, and you lapsed back into complaints and criticism. I'm wondering if we could look at how you each might have been feeling after talking so openly and honestly.

Being able to identify my own reactions and empathize with them without necessarily having to know the origins of those reactions in that moment helped me disclose rather than disconnect. Often this disclosure facilitated their return to more authentic sharing, and they would venture into the risky waters of revealing how much fear accompanied the possibility of getting what they so desperately wanted.

OWNERSHIP OF FEELINGS AND
SELF–OTHER DIFFERENTIATION

As our trust in one another deepened, and as they came to better understand the various steps to their relational dances of brief connection–disconnection–stronger connection in a depathologized way, they made slow but steady progress in their awareness of, and willingness to expose, disavowed parts of themselves. This area of growth was facilitated by several external events that temporarily restressed the pair and challenged—but then strengthened—their tenuous connection. For example, they precipitously lost several child-care workers one after another—an experience that provided numerous opportunities for them to practice authentic sharing and disclosure of genuine expectations, as well as a chance to resist a return to the old pattern in which Elise "picked up the slack" and suffered bitterly in silence. A vacation that involved Mick meeting a woman friend from his past for the day precipitated powerful feelings of betrayal, jealousy, and envy in Elise—all of which were very difficult feelings for her to admit to herself, let alone to Mick. Eventually she risked tentatively exposing these feelings to Mick and then struggled to identify what she might need from him to repair the hurt. I consistently shared my pride in her courage, yet had to titrate my enthusiasm carefully, because she was still very uncomfortable receiving support and "too much" often triggered a disconnect.

Around this time, Elise took several trips home, which enabled her to plan and then practice new strategies for connecting with her mother. I reminded Elise about the dynamic of the relational paradox—that her yearnings for connection to her mother still felt dangerous and sensitized her to want to disconnect from her mother, usually through silence, shame, and pseudo-compliance. Both sides of the paradox needed our acknowledgment and respect; although her mother has deeply wounded her, she is also someone Elise continued to need. Understanding the paradox in relation to her mother opened the way for her to think of Mick in a similar fashion. We were then able to talk more about the ways in which we are all flawed and that it is possible to be hurt by someone we also love and badly need. For example, Mick had long idealized Elise's mother, soliciting her attention and advice and regularly pointing out to Elise how much he enjoyed her mother's company. Elise, who felt a mix of critical guilt and shame for her negative feelings toward her mother, was outwardly unresponsive to Mick but deeply hurt. Slowly, she persisted in voicing her truth and clarifying her unique experiences with her mother, which were very different from Mick's experiences with her as his mother-in-law, and this differentiation enhanced Elise's feelings of success, empowerment, and vitality. She also surprisingly (to her) felt closer to Mick as a result.

Another critical juncture occurred several months later as they were hovering on the precipice of deeper sharing and risk taking. They diverted themselves with conflicts about child management. Elise had recently fired their 12-year-old son's individual therapist, saying that she had more trust in my opinion and wondered if they should bring him to our sessions. I responded that perhaps they were feeling readier to work together as a couple to manage their son's risky and frightening behavior. For weeks, they brought in assorted problems about their son, and I chose to help them examine the mutual struggle from the perspective of the relational paradox and what they already knew about their respective strategies of disconnection. Since I regularly see families, and the issue was another opportunity to increase their sense of empowerment (this time, as parents), I found it challenging to decide whether to include their son or continue to help them develop a stronger parenting alliance in the couple format. Elise, in particular, found it very difficult to expose her uncertainties about her mothering as well as identify her points of difference with Mick. Maintaining the emphasis on the couple facilitated her ability to share many deep doubts she later stated she would have found difficult to expose with their son in attendance. Furthermore, understanding our sessions as a time in which they gathered their courage and confidence to move deeper allowed them to recognize (after several weeks) that they were "getting away from what they came to do." This realization was followed by a critical awareness for Elise that, during the course of their relationship, she had been trying to help Mick by making him more like her, instead of "really listening to what he truly needed." She then understood her frustration in a new way.

To every juncture, I attempted to bring my curiosity and view of the impasse/struggle as an opportunity for authentic expression, self–other differentiation, and connection.

REWORKING RELATIONAL IMAGES, ASSERTING SELF IN RELATIONSHIP DIFFERENTLY, AND CONNECTING ACROSS DIFFERENCE

The key relational themes that informed the processes of therapy revolved around the relational images of emotional impoverishment and isolation in the histories of both Mick and Elise. Although the core images were similar, I found it important throughout our work to highlight both the similarities and the differences in the coping strategies they each had developed. For example, Mick's early family experiences of loss left him feeling that it was unsafe to get close to anyone because the person would surely leave or hurt him. He alternated between feeling that he did not deserve anything better and frantically trying to make Elise and others give him what he needed (by being Mr. Nice Guy "I'll be so good you'll have to comply," etc.). Elise's early family experiences of emotional neglect taught her that it is safer not to need ("I'm a perfect superwoman") than to risk the pain and despair of asking and being disappointed. Therefore, Elise chose not to need anything from Mick, who needed to be needed.

Mick's Relational Image: "There Is Not Enough to Go Around—I Must Work Very Hard to Be the Best and Worthiest of Attention"

Mick regularly put himself in a one-down position in relation to Elise professionally (e.g., she made more money, did more difficult work, etc.), then would double his efforts to be the best dad or take on extra household responsibilities in misguided attempts to earn her attention and respect, even while losing self-respect in the process. One of the most distressing ways they had devised to manage the competitive feelings in the relationship was to almost totally separate their work lives. Gradually, they had stopped going to each other's social functions from their respective workplaces, had withheld and/or tightly guarded information about work personalities and events, and had almost totally stopped using one another as a supportive ear for the normal ups and downs of their professional lives. Elise would comment: "I can't possibly tell him that I got x award or tell him how much I love what I do because he doesn't want to hear it." Likewise, Mick found Elise unsympathetic toward his work problems and "uninterested" in the staff, whom he "loved." Neither believed the other to be genuinely concerned about what they devoted so much time and attention to, because they were convinced the other took their success as a personal affront. I regularly reflected my genuine feelings of concern at the ways they were excluding each other from such an important and vital aspect of their relationship. It appeared to be very difficult for them to accept my regular invitations to risk sharing some piece of information about their work lives. They each strongly believed that the other would be "too hurt if I told the truth." I responded that I saw the chronic disengagement around work to already be very hurtful—and both Mick and Elise admitted that was true. As Mick began to implement and sustain the small changes in controlling his weekly schedule, he began to experience some relief from the anxiety. Ever so slowly, he also began to feel some successes at work, which he then shared with Elise. She was relieved and pleased to be included and slowly was more able to respond with more encouragement for Mick as well as with several examples from her own professional experience. Much riskier was the process of beginning to identify and examine how personal feelings of failure/imperfection could be experienced as belonging to the other. For example, when

Mick was feeling most discouraged about his performance, he was likely to criticize Elise for failing to show interest in his problems. I tried to stay connected to my belief that watching for, and then building upon, opportunities to clarify the feelings of self versus other helped them become more empathic and open to deepening their connection.

Another example of their competitiveness was apparent in the ways they responded to, and used, me in our sessions. Mick was exquisitely sensitive to the degree of attention I afforded him, particularly when distressed, and was inevitably disappointed when I encouraged Elise to come more and more into her voice. If I spent "too much time" (in his eyes) focused on Elise, he would either withdraw into a pout, interrupt, or silently communicate extreme irritation. Responding to him felt delicate; sometimes he would be open to my challenging observations, but at other times he would retreat further. Once his reactivity became manageable enough to allow me to focus on Elise, and once Elise, ever so slowly, grew more able to tolerate attention as well as speak up, Mick began to hear things he did not particularly like. It was at this point that he began phoning me between sessions. I realized that Mick's relational image at play here was the one that developed with his mother: "I will be your good and special little boy in return for special, exclusive treatment from you." I was challenging that dynamic by encouraging Elise to speak out honestly about her reactions toward him as well as by countering his efforts to disconnect from the deepening couple work. His calls were infrequent (once every 3–6 weeks), short in length, and usually centered around his wanting me to know something "from his perspective," to take the opportunity to more fully react to something that had been said in the previous session or to inform me of a comment Elise had made at home that he "knew she wouldn't bring up." This was all done in an innocuous tone of voice, implying "I'm just trying to be helpful."

At first, I indulged his calls with brief responses. Then, when I tried to cut him short, always with the recommendation that what he was sharing was very important to bring into the session together, I usually felt brushed off, as though I had not fully appreciate how helpful he was trying to be. Usually, he did not take my recommendation to bring the outside contact into the session, and, of course, I felt "caught" between the two of them. I spent time puzzling about what was behind my atypical lapse of directness for these kinds of situations. I knew that one of my relational images of gaining special status by good behavior was being evoked—a part of me liked the specialness created by believing that I could better respond to Mick, do a better job of meeting his needs, than Elise. To what extent was I trying to keep this exclusivity between Mick and me alive? I felt both pleased by the contacts and uncomfortable with my pleasure. I decided that I needed to bring up my discomfort and genu-

ine concern about the impact of these outside contacts on their relationship and the alliance between us. Then, the following event happened.

Mick came to the session appearing quite depressed and distant, and
Elise looked confused and somewhat frightened. Both remarked that they
had had a "bad week," had several circular fights about "stupid shit,"
which left them feeling "like we can't hold onto what we're doing here."
Mick expressed considerable hurt around his perception that Elise just
"refused to see" how hard he was trying to be helpful and mentioned several aborted attempts to be helpful to her (one of which I heard as an
oblique reference to something I had coached him, in a phone contact, to
bring to the session). Viewing this set of circumstances as the opportunity
I had been waiting for, I asked Mick to describe that hurt feeling. While
sharing the very first incident that week in which he felt "slighted," he began to cry and the details became hazy. He was totally absorbed in the
pain of remembering what was clearly not just something that had happened that week. As he cried, Elise reached over and touched his arm—
something she had never done in more than 10 months of therapy—and
his sobbing deepened. I asked if he would be willing to travel back in time
in his mind to an earlier moment when he could remember having this
particular feeling. He put his hand over his heart and talked about the
many times, as a young boy and adolescent, he had listened to his parents
fighting and felt "sick in his belly." He would listen for his father to storm
off, then wait for the moment to come downstairs to comfort his mother,
often ministering to her bruises and cuts. One time, he went to "help" his
mother, not realizing that his father had not left the house. As his whole
body shook, Mick described his father "coming from out of nowhere" and
screaming at Mick to "get the hell out of here" and to "quit coming between" them. Hitting Mick, he also pushed his wife out of the room, while
restraining Mick from going to her. Mick described desperately trying to
make his father understand, to find a way to get back in his good graces,
but he was left instead with days of punishing isolation. "Worst of all, my
mother kept her distance from me, and I could barely stand that."

I felt deeply moved by Mick's pain and by Elise's small display of comfort to him. I asked if she had known about this story, and she said she
had heard different examples of how bad it got but had "no idea it could
have affected Mick like this." Mick then shared how guilty he felt (feels)
that he was not able to keep his mother alive—that he could not help her
create a better life with his father and that (irrationally) he could not keep
her from having the stroke that killed her. I responded that I could imagine what it must have been like to feel as though he had to be so good and
helpful all the time to compete for his parents' affection, only to be abandoned by both, over and over again. As his crying subsided and his whole

body softened, he made the connection that he gets to a point with Elise where he "can't stand feeling alone anymore," that he "feels like a needy ass who keeps trying to get something but never gets it and just feels bad for wanting it."

We talked together about how that pattern would unfold between them: how Elise would miss his signals but sense his disconnection. He was able to say that he "felt so strongly that he should get it" (i.e., attention). I asked if he ever felt that way in our sessions. He said that he guessed he did, especially when he felt that neither of us "really got what he was trying to say." I asked what he did at those times, and Mick took the leap, sharing that "a couple times, I called you." Elise looked surprised but listened attentively as he described the helpless, shameful feelings associated with loneliness and how he "just was trying to help." We identified a need for Elise to learn how to better read his signals, and I pointed out that her empathic presence in this session—her ability to be with him in the moment—demonstrated that she could, in fact, tolerate his neediness. I attempted to ally with the helpful part of him to build awareness that the outside calling was one of those examples when "good intentions" could have problematic consequences for the relationship as well as for our ability to work together successfully. At that session and in the future, I did my best to find a variety of ways to express the following message repeatedly:

> "Mick, I know how much you want Elise to understand and appreciate you, and I know how much Elise wants to meet your needs. This is a place for each of you to stretch, to risk and grow. Your risk is to bring up to her what you are afraid she cannot hear, and her risk will be to do her very best to hear and respond to you, knowing that her response may not always suffice. Bringing your feelings to her is much more important than bringing them to me privately, although I will be here to help you each try and connect as well as to try and understand why connection may not be possible at that moment."

Fortunately, we were able to reference that mutually empowering session in the future and access a different, present-day relational image that was less bleak. Eventually, Mick developed an appreciation that disappointment and fear can be tolerated and that it is more meaningful to speak authentically and to feel understood and responded to than having to always "get what I want in the way I want it." Over time, Elise learned to protect Mick less and to identify ways she might be more appropriately self-protective.

Elise's Relational Image: "Neediness and Vulnerability Are Imperfections and 'Shameful' and Cause Others to Abandon Me"

Elise was much more guarded and less open not only about her competitiveness but also about herself, in general. She had a picture of herself as the all-knowing "superwoman" who needed nothing from anyone but could perfectly meet the needs of everyone around her. She exuded an aura that suggested "I am above competition." This attitude was highly offensive to Mick, of course, and he had a difficult time believing that she was essentially unconscious of the ways in which she came across to others. When it became more "acceptable" to talk openly about their work, Elise shared that she knew she was intimidating to colleagues but she "put up with that" because she never doubted that they all respected her. She could "live with being feared but could not live with not being viewed as the best." She "never had time to waste worrying about what other people thought of her—there was too much important work to be done." It never occurred to her that she did not leave that demeanor at work but carried it with her through the door every night.

During one session she was able to admit to feeling frustrated by my regular invitations to her to identify what it was that she wanted/needed, saying, "I have absolutely no clue what that is—how can I ask for it?" I wondered aloud if a change in our structure to include individual sessions might not help her explore and focus on the identification of her needs (particularly since Mick was, at this point, more able to "share the spotlight"). Frequently, in the context of a couple treatment, I will do intense pieces of work with one partner while the other bears witness to that work. But because Elise was having such a difficult time expressing herself (particularly if she felt her feelings would challenge Mick), I thought that offering several individual sessions might increase her trust in me and her comfort level, which would help her risk bringing more of herself into the sessions. At first, she withdrew into silence, then slowly shared her fear of the change, since she "counted on the couple sessions so much" to teach her to speak up and to feel some connection with Mick. Her statement strongly touched Mick, and he was able to reassure her about his commitment to the work and to encourage her to "learn to take some attention." He was even able to say that he believed her ability to take more in would also help their relationship. She expressed appreciation but was clearly not ready to make the change.

Several sessions later, we were talking about an incident that had occurred during the week in which she failed to pick up their son on time and how critical she felt of herself. After numerous attempts at empathy that seemed to fall on deaf ears, I was feeling particularly frustrated by my inability to reach her. I began to share an example from my own struggles with perfection—my attempts to meet everyone else's needs but my own. Though she remained quiet, I felt her intensely connected and appreciative. Ever so slowly, and in response to my regular efforts to communicate my patience with her need to protect herself by sharing my ongoing struggles with the same controlling images and self-expectations, she began to talk about how good it felt to be able to "take in some help." She also began to describe "how lonely it felt at the top" and how she really did not want others to experience her as aloof and uncaring—particularly Mick. Similarly, Mick began to talk about the picture he had of himself as humorously "leading with his (physical) disabilities" and how his self-presentation was designed to keep people away from his authentic feelings of humiliation and shame. He wondered if perhaps because he had developed a capacity to expose neediness and be the proverbial squeaky wheel, he had come to believe that he was "more open than Elise." Elise was visibly touched by this exchange and at the end of the session asked if we could begin to have some individual sessions.

Being able to talk about how all of us subscribed to this cult of self-sufficiency—in essence, "the less I need and the more I can do for myself, the better person I am"—was mutually freeing. We each shared ways in which our own personal sense of isolation could turn into a breeding ground of struggles to gain positions of superiority with colleagues, friends, and family. Regularly naming this trap and putting it outside of us detoxified its effects and encouraged positive acts of resistance and resilience.

I strongly identified with Mick and Elise's key relational strategy to focus on healing others in a partial attempt to heal the self. I knew that much of my motivation to help others, first as a nurse, then as a clinical psychologist, was an effort to assuage my guilt over my inability to keep my beloved mother alive. It was a way of keeping her with me but also a way of keeping parts of myself trapped in servitude to an impossible goal. I found that the more I was able to bring my own struggle, which was a variant of each of theirs, into the room and name the ways in which those efforts both moved us toward and away from connection, the levels of mutual authenticity and risk taking intensified and the sense of our collective humanity deepened.

CURRENT STATUS

Mick and Elise are midway into their second year of therapy. Our process has been greatly facilitated by the mutual determination both partners bring to the change effort. They had the financial resources and were willing to commit the time to come for regular sessions. Although getting them to commit to between-session homework and devote additional time to the relationship has been much more difficult and sporadic, they have taken increasing responsibility for actively participating in moving the therapy forward. The general lack of external constraints allowed them to proceed at the slow pace they required to build safety and trust and to work their way through the spiral of deepening authenticity and connection.

After my initial suggestion to supplement couple work with individual sessions with Elise, my ambivalence resurfaced. I believe in the value of witnessing; just as Elise needed to learn more about her own feelings and how to articulate them, Mick needed to learn ways to empathically resonate with those feelings. But my instincts were telling me we had been hovering on a plateau, and that helping Elise to bring in more of herself would stimulate a positive shift. I thought the individual sessions might be useful in furthering the work in relation to Elise's relational image of a critical/unresponsive mother. I believed Elise could greatly benefit from becoming aware of, and being able to express and examine, her feelings with a curious, nurturing, and empathic listener (hopefully, me). Yet I was also concerned that individual sessions with Elise might trigger a flight into competition between Mick and Elise over my attention and diminish their growing intimacy.

Currently, we have weekly couple sessions, and Elise and I have had three supplemental individual sessions. We are in agreement that this structure seems to be providing a "good enough" holding and is subject to regular evaluations. Elise appears to be more comfortable with the "real spotlight," as she has come to call it (to distinguish it from the pseudo-spotlight she has more typically held). She is beginning to develop an appreciation for the way in which her belief that she must "do it all" helps Mick believe that she does not, in fact, need or want anything—which, in turn, backfires on them both. I know that she knows I have a deep understanding of, and respect for, that part of her that believes that if she let go of one little detail, her world (she) could collapse and no one would be there to help. She knows that I admire her courage and find it mutually empowering. When she challenges these relational images, for example, by asking for help from Mick or me or revealing her feelings of uncertainty, I feel encouraged and reenergized to take similar risks in my own relationships, including with them.

She has just begun to ask about the pragmatics of how I manage a dual-career lifestyle and allow herself to be moved (humorously and otherwise) by a story or two of my own disasters. She has begun to bring in examples of times when she holds back a request for something she wants from Mick, and although it feels familiar to do so, it is also "personally costly to me and us." Additionally reassuring is the fact that the couple sessions have become reinvigorated: Elise is bringing more of herself into the relationship, and Mick is increasingly able to listen, reflect, and respond to who she is in the moment, not who he needs her to be. The image (the "we") they recently offered for their current relationship is:

> "We're like the big pot we just bought [for the garden]—sturdy, showy, and solid on the outside, but when you look in, there is another container that is plexiglass with colorful designs that you need to handle carefully because it is breakable and not as tough as it looks. But it is an interesting pot—more than meets the eye!"

At the same time, Mick and Elise are gaining clarity about, and grieving for, who they thought each other was and the way the relationship had been organized to maintain those relational images and illusions. They are struggling to identify what they really need for themselves and what they are willing to do to get it. Although each is better able to feel more in the presence of the other, doing so remains a delicate process because both feel more frightened than when they started therapy, that once the other "truly" knows who they are and what they need, then they will be abandoned and the marriage will fail. The ongoing fuel nourishing their courage is the mutual empowerment each feels in the safety and trust developed in the truth-telling therapy encounters.

REFERENCES

Jordan, J. (1992). Relational resilience. *Work in Progress, No. 57.* Wellesley, MA: Stone Center Working Paper Series.

Jordan, J. (1995). Relational awareness: Transforming disconnection. *Work in Progress, No. 76.* Wellesley, MA: Stone Center Working Paper Series.

Madsen, W. C. (1999). *Collaborative therapy with multi-stressed families: From old problems to new futures.* New York: Guilford Press.

Miller, J. B. (2001). *Change in therapy.* Paper presented at a symposium at the Jean Baker Miller Advanced Summer Training Institute, Wellesley, MA.

Miller, J. B., & Stiver, I. P. (1997). *The healing connection.* Boston: Beacon Press.

Nemiroff, R., & Colarusso, C. (1990). *New dimensions in adult development.* New York: Basic Books.

Real, T. (1997). *I don't want to talk about it.* New York: Scribner.

Sharpe, S. A. (2000). *The ways we love: A developmental approach to treating couples.* New York: Guilford Press.

Shem, S., & Surrey, J. (1998). *We have to talk.* New York: Basic Books.

Skerrett, K. (1996). From isolation to mutuality: A feminist collaborative model of couples therapy. *Women and Therapy, 19*(3), 93–106.

Skerrett, K. (1997). Women's development in the family: A thematic view. *Journal of Feminist Family Therapy, 9*(4), 15–41.

Skerrett, K. (2003). Couple dialogues with illness: Expanding the "We." *Families, Systems and Health, 21*(1), 49–60.

Weingarten, K. (1991). The discourses of intimacy: Adding a social constructionist and feminist view. *Family Process, 30*, 285–305.

9

The Five Good Things
in Cross-Cultural Therapy

ROSEANN ADAMS

> To the extent that we are unable to speak with authenticity
> about conflict, power, and race, we become caught in the
> grip of shame where historical hurts can override our most
> genuine yearnings for connection.
> —MAUREEN WALKER (1999, p. 5)

*S*uccessful therapeutic engagement between white therapists and black clients challenges traditional approaches to psychotherapy. Many established models of practice are based on theories of human behavior that reflect European and Anglo American culture. Research on cross-cultural psychotherapy (using traditional models) has found that there is a high likelihood of client dropout in black–white therapist–client dyads (Sue, 1977; Sue, McKinney, Allen, & Hall, 1974). Black clients generally attend fewer sessions than white clients (Gwyn & Kilpatrick, 1981). Cross-cultural psychotherapy conducted under unexamined Eurocentric values is less likely to be a positive and growth-producing experience for either client or therapist.

Relational–cultural theory is based on a philosophy of cultural pluralism in which differences between people, especially cultural differences, are viewed as important. The theory's focus on the interaction between macro issues and micro problems makes it an especially effective approach for cross-cultural clinical work. In such work, the therapist must recognize and manage issues that might inhibit both therapist and client.

151

Maureen Walker (1999) has described the "grip of shame" as a force that prevents the possibility of authentic connection. Yet by acknowledging, naming, and examining the impact of conflict, power, race, and culture on both therapist and client, it is possible to loosen that grip of shame that Walker describes. A new, more authentic relationship can then be created.

Relational–cultural theory has increased both my awareness of, and my ability to examine the impact of, power, race, and culture in all of my clinical work. This new awareness has been especially helpful in my work with clients who are members of marginalized groups. As the daughter of working-class immigrant parents, I do not easily see myself as standing on the higher rungs of the white social hierarchy in this country. I am much more comfortable taking the position as sister and ally to the oppressed than I am in examining how I derive benefits from my unearned white privilege. As a well-meaning, well-intentioned, liberal white therapist, I am at risk not only of minimizing, ignoring, or misunderstanding the impact of cultural difference but of making too much of it. I am also at risk of missing, denying, or avoiding the naming of racism in its subtle and painful everyday expressions.

In relational–cultural theory, psychological growth is viewed as occurring in and through relationships with others. Both identity of self and understanding of others are formed through relationships and through a history of interactional patterns in relational experiences (Miller & Stiver, 1998). Authenticity is described as "the ability to put forward feelings and thoughts . . . and to stand by them" (p. 30). "Mutual empathy" occurs when each person is heard, understood, and accepted. When mutual empathy is established in a relational connection, each person is encouraged to bring more and more of his or her authentic self into relationship. When thoughts and feelings are not heard, understood, or responded to empathically, mutual empathy cannot develop and disconnection occurs. This relationship dynamic results in the formation of relational images that predict disconnection. The person learns to anticipate that authentic expression of self will result in isolation, devaluation, and disconnection. Repeated experiences of disconnection reinforce and elaborate relational images that portray others as potential perpetrators of personal injury.

A history of separation and abuse of power shapes the relational images that black and whites have of each other. Experiences of racism, prejudice, and discrimination lead to the development of strategies for disconnection that support the illusion of safety. As a result, members of black–white therapist–client dyads may present less than authentic versions of themselves to each other, especially in the important initial contacts. For example, a black person who is open, responsive, and expressive in interactions with other blacks may be quiet, reserved, formal, and distant in initial interactions with a white therapist. The white therapist, in turn, may feel restricted by fear of exposing his or her deficiencies in cultural competence and may feel inhibited by racial guilt. As a white therapist with black clients, I have recognized moments when my discomfort acknowledging difference has limited my capacity to be authentic, genuine, and emotionally available. On those occasions, my effectiveness as a therapist is diminished.

An essential ongoing aspect of the work for the relational–cultural therapist in cross-cultural therapy is taking responsibility for the co-creation of a context of safety within a racially unsafe culture. This context of safety enables both client and therapist to continuously bring more of the authentic self into the room and into the relationship. If a therapeutic alliance with a black client awaits creation, then it is up to the white therapist to open a space to explore the positive and negative relational images the client has of whites, per se, and specifically of whites "helping others." The white therapist must strive to be conscious of, and honest about, his or her relational images of blacks and black–white relationships and examine how those images may limit or enlarge the capacity to be authentic, to genuinely feel and express empathy in ways that the client can understand and accept.

Direction and guidance obtained through continuing education, clinical supervision, and consultation are essential resources that support growth in competence in cross-cultural work. While striving toward cultural competence is an important goal, it is also important to humbly recognize our (the therapist's) own not knowing and the need for client and therapist to collaboratively develop an understanding of the client's life and relationships. Balancing study toward an ever-elusive goal of cultural competence with acceptance and acknowledgment of the limitations of our competence requires ongoing support. For me, that direction and guidance come from several sources: most significantly, the faculty and fellow students of relational–cultural theory, whom I have met through my affiliation with the Jean Baker Miller Training Institute; my colleagues at Cathedral Counseling Center and the Chicago Association for the Advancement of Relational–Cultural Theory; the faculty of the Chicago Center for Family Health; and staff members of the Illinois Department of Children and Family Services.

As a result of social change, blacks and whites may have more experiences working in the same places, going to the same schools, shopping in the same stores, and eating in the same restaurants. However, it may be that *separate but equal* has been exchanged with a subtler and more confusing *same place, different section*—or what Steinhorn and Diggs-Brown (1999) have described as the "illusion of integration." For the most part, blacks and whites continue to live socially and emotionally segregated lives. We celebrate life's joys, grieve life's sorrows, share our private thoughts, and express our deep longings most often with people who live on our own side of the great racial divide. The challenge of the relational–cultural therapist doing cross-cultural clinical work is that of creating a relationship that empowers both client and therapist to stretch across that vast divide and connect—to see each other, hear each other, understand each other, and be moved by, with, and toward each other.

CLINICAL CASE EXAMPLE

Until recently, much of the published clinical case material demonstrating the application of relational–cultural theory presented examples of individual long-term treatment between white women clients and their white women therapists. The therapeutic relationship described in this chapter demonstrates the practical application of relational–cultural theory in a clinical case that has three distinguishing features: (1) a context of managed care short-term treatment (18 sessions over the course of 7 months); (2) family rather than individual as client; and (3) cross-cultural dynamic of white therapist with black family.

This story of my work with the Smith family, told in my voice and from my perspective, is a reflection of my experience of the relationship. The family generously gave me permission to tell the story of our work together. The names, facts, and identifying information have been changed to protect the family's anonymity.

First Contact

My story with the Smith family began with a phone call. Mrs. Smith contacted her health insurance company to obtain names of therapists who work with families and who are willing to schedule evening or Saturday appointments. She left me a voice-mail message stating that she needed to see someone about her 11-year-old stepdaughter and that she wanted to schedule an appointment as soon as possible. One of the things I have learned over the years is the importance of responding promptly to a client's first call. Clients who get a response to their first call within 24 hours are much more likely to schedule a first appointment. I returned Mrs. Smith's call within a few hours of picking up her message, contacting her at her office phone number. In our first conversation, Mrs. Smith put me on hold several times while she took a series of incoming calls. My initial reaction was irritation with what I experienced as her disrespect for my time. The truth, however, is that I was calling her at a time that was convenient for me, and that time may not have been the most convenient for her.

Unacknowledged, unnamed, and unexamined power differentials and imbalances create the greatest potential for disconnection and violation in therapy. Mental health service delivery models are typically based on a hierarchical power structure, in which the person who asks for help is in a one-down, less powerful position. The application of relational–cultural theory to cross-cultural treatment requires that the therapist maintain "ongoing active attention to his or her own personal internalized dominance and oppression" (Jenkins, 2000, p. 8). The goal for the relational–cultural therapist is not to ignore or deny differences in power and authority but rather to be aware of how those differences lead the therapist to act in relationship and to understand how power and authority can be used most respectfully on behalf of him- or herself, the client, and the therapeutic relationship.

Mrs. Smith told me that she had been forced to "jump through too many hoops" with her insurance company just to get a few names. She said she had called three other people, and no one had called her back. We spent a few minutes on the phone while she explained that she was newly married with two young sons from a prior relationship. Her husband recently announced his wish to have his 11-year-old daughter from a previous relationship come to live with his new family. Mrs. Smith described her stepdaughter as disobedient and manipulative and asked if I would be able to meet with the child the next day. I explained that I would want to schedule a first appointment with her and her husband to discuss how I could be most helpful to them before meeting with her stepdaughter. Mrs. Smith said she did not think that would work and she did not understand why I needed to see her and her husband if the problem was with the child.

Observations and assessments are part of the therapy process. Throughout the course of therapy, the therapist is not the only person making observations and formulating assessments. The client (be it individual, couple, or family), is making an assessment of value regarding the services offered and formulating an evaluation of the therapist to determine if the required financial expense, physical and emotional effort, and investment of time will result in something beneficial for them. Whenever I begin a new therapy relationship, I remind myself that it is up to me, especially in the first few meetings but also throughout the length of the relationship, to provide a context in which clients feel hope that the moments we spend together in my office will make a positive difference in their "real" world, their everyday lives, and in the quality of their relationships. The first few contacts are crucial in establishing the foundation of trust for ongoing work. For people who have never been in therapy, both the process and the person of the therapist may be initially difficult to trust. A cross-cultural dynamic further complicates the process.

In working with families, it is important to communicate a respect for the parents' rights to evaluate and choose the help for themselves and their children that they deem beneficial. Meeting with parents before meeting with children gives parents the opportunity to determine whether *they* feel comfortable enough with me to trust me with their children. In two-parent heterosexual families, fathers are frequently not treated as essential members in family therapy. Most often it is the mother who makes the call to the therapist, and it is she who schedules the first appointment. My experience is that treatment is often more effective when an alliance is developed with both parents in a two-parent family. In Mrs. Smith's case, I also heard that she was feeling overwhelmed. In most cases, women take the greatest share of the burden in caring for children. If Mr. Smith had not been encouraged to come to the session, there would be less opportunity for Mrs. Smith to accept help and support from her husband in caring for their family. I wanted to do whatever I could to begin the treatment by facilitating the potential for establishing a partnership with both parents. Mrs. Smith had only recently gotten to know her new stepdaughter, Kinesha. Mr. Smith's perspective on Kinesha's behavior and knowledge of her history would likely be helpful to us. I described some of these reasons for wanting to have the first meeting with both parents and expressed empathy with Mrs. Smith's desire to get help for her stepdaughter.

Mrs. Smith said she would talk to her husband and call me back. Two days later Mrs. Smith left me another message, asking for an appointment for herself and her husband and suggesting several times and dates that would work for them. I returned her call, and we confirmed an appointment time for the next week. I explained the fee arrangements and let her know that she needed to bring her insurance card and a certification for services from the insurance company. I said that it would be best if she and her husband could come to the first meeting without the children, because the children might have a hard time waiting while the three of us met. She told me that her children were well behaved, and if she was not able to get someone to watch them at home, she would just have to bring them. On the day of the appointment, I met Janet and Robert Smith, Robert's 11-year-old daughter Kinesha, and Janet's two sons, James, 9, and David, 7.

The First Session

Many times my clients refer to themselves and other clients as "customers." In bringing the children to the first appointment, Janet was inviting me to reconsider my way of serving clients with children. If families with young children are my customers, serving them well not only requires that I schedule appointments during their nonworking hours but also that I consider ways to make my services more accessible for parents by accommodating and welcoming their children.

Thinking about providing therapy as a *service* to my clients, *who are my customers*, has changed how I respond to verbal and behavioral client communications that would be more traditionally considered expressions of "resistance." In relational–cultural theory, concepts of *mutuality* and *mutual empathy* (Jordan, 1991) describe relational processes that foster growth, connection, and transformation. As Jordan (1991) states:

> A model that recognizes that therapy is a dialogue also recognizes that therapy is characterized by a process of mutual change and impact. Both therapist and patient are touched emotionally by each other, grow in relationship, gain something from one another, risk something of themselves in the process . . . in short, both are affected, changed, part of an open system of feeling and learning. There is significant mutuality. It takes courage on both sides to involve themselves in this interaction. (p. 288)

Giving attention to the process of mutual empathy leads me to be more open to hearing how my clients experience our interactions, and as a result, I am more open to being moved and influenced by what I hear and see—to consider changing what I do and how I do it, based on the client's experiences.

Janet was a petite, light-skinned woman who was dressed in a business suit. Dressed in jeans and a polo shirt, Robert, at over 6 feet tall, towered over Janet. Janet's boys were small, thin, neatly dressed, and extremely polite. Kinesha was dark-skinned, tall like her father, and, in contrast to the rest of the family, looked somewhat disheveled. She was dressed in sweatpants and a sweatshirt that fit her poorly and had several large stains and tears in the knees and the elbows. Each of the two boys carried backpacks containing books, paper, markers, and juice boxes and snacks. Kinesha had no backpack or books or snacks. I asked her if she liked to draw, and I gave her some paper and crayons. The waiting room had no place for Kinesha to sit comfortably while she drew. In an effort to attend to Kinesha in the therapeutic context, I rearranged some furniture in the waiting room to create a more comfortable place for her to sit and draw. I silently noted the physical differences between Kinesha and Janet and how the boys looked so much more cared for than did Kinesha. I wondered how Janet and Kinesha felt about the physical differences between them (skin color, hair texture, body type) and how those differences influenced their relationship. I also wondered about the difference in the evidence of being cared for among the children.

After getting the children settled in the waiting room, I showed Janet and Robert to my office. Successful beginnings in clinical work are dependent upon the therapist's ability to communicate humanity, warmth, concern, caring, respect, and honesty in ways that match the client's vision and definition of those qualities. Confusion about the contrived nature or artificial quality of therapist–client relationship may inhibit the potential for authentic interaction and impede the creation of a real person-to-person human connection. Therapist speech and body language that convey a genuine message of welcome can strongly influence the client's decision about whether or not to continue treatment. I greeted the Smiths and let them know they could call me by my first name, and I asked them how they preferred to be addressed. Both the Smiths asked to be called by their first names. I summarized what I understood of the family situation from what I had learned in the first phone call with Janet and thanked them both for coming. I asked them if they had anything that would add to my understanding of what was happening in their family. Robert spoke first. He said that he did not think Kinesha or anyone in the family needed therapy. He said he agreed to come because he knew Janet was having a hard time with Kinesha, and he wanted to do whatever he could to help Janet and Kinesha get along better so that they could all live together. I responded to his question about the family's need for therapy by saying something about how our work together might be helpful in supporting their goal of blending their two families. I thanked him for coming and said that since he was the person who probably knew Kinesha best, I was glad that we would have the benefit of his impressions.

I explained that I wanted to get the necessary paperwork out of the way first and then we could discuss what brought them in and how I might be helpful to them. I asked Janet for the insurance card and certification for treatment form. Janet apologized for having neither item, explaining that she had left her office in a hurry in order to get home and get the children ready. Janet described the family's frantic rush as Robert had arrived late from picking Kinesha up from her mother's. In the family's dash to arrive on time, the insurance papers had been left on the kitchen table. She said she could either drop the forms off the next day or mail them to me. Robert defended himself against Janet's comment about his being late by explaining that he had taken longer because he had spent time trying, unsuccessfully, to convince Kinesha to change her clothes, anticipating his wife's negative reaction to his daughter's appearance. This interaction over insurance forms provided me with some information about the difference between Kenisha's clothing and grooming and that of her younger stepbrothers. In an effort at being empathic with Janet's stress, I commented that it must have been difficult to rush from her office, get everyone ready and drive back downtown for a meeting to which nobody was looking forward. I told Janet that it would be fine to either mail the forms or bring them to the next meeting. In working with managed care, the completion of forms can be a time-consuming and complicated process. I like to discuss the forms with clients and begin the process of completing requests for additional sessions as early as possible to build in leeway for the lengthy response time so that treatment is not interrupted while we wait for additional sessions to be approved.

Neither Janet nor Robert had ever seen a therapist before, so we talked about logistics, length of our meetings, and frequency of sessions. I have found that the traditional 50-minute hour is not always the best for couple or family sessions. Scheduling 75- or 90-minute sessions allows each person ample opportunity to speak and leaves the family feeling that the meeting was long enough to have been worth the time and trouble required to get there. Families with young children are often stressed by rushing from one place to another. Sometimes a willingness to schedule longer sessions and/or meeting less frequently than once a week can communicate an appreciation for the family's real-life demands and an openness to accommodate the busy schedule. Offering flexibility in scheduling appointments enables family members to allocate time for therapy in a way that works best for them and reduces the likelihood of missed or failed appointments. My willingness to be flexible in scheduling both frequency and length of sessions was greatly appreciated by the Smith family and contributed to our ability to establish a positive, cooperative working relationship. Most of the time they preferred scheduling our appointments so that sessions were at least 75 minutes long, and we met less frequently than once each week.

I explained to the Smiths that I would be asking them questions to learn about them and their children and that if, at anytime, they felt uncomfortable with my questions, to please let me know. I often feel pushed by the length of treatment limitations imposed by managed care. My own anxiety about getting as much done in as little time as possible can result in the client feeling interrogated, as I hurry to collect information about family history and presenting problems. Sensitivity to the client's experience of the information-gathering process is especially important in cross-cultural work in terms of establishing a context of mutual trust and empathy. Boyd-Franklin (2003) identifies the potential danger of the black family's early termination from treatment as a result of feeling that the white therapist is "prying into their business" before trust has been established. Sensitivity to the possibility of the family's past negative experiences with social institutions and agencies and the family's fear of exposing secrets that might be used against them requires that the therapist proceed with respect and patience in allowing details and factual information to unfold over the course of the therapy.

When I asked the couple to describe how things were going with them, Janet spoke first. She said she was feeling overwhelmed following the couple's recent marriage. She felt burdened by the demands of three children, pushed by increased demands at work due to her recent promotion, stressed by financial pressures, and disorganized by the family's move to a new apartment. Her husband's recent announcement that he wanted Kinesha to live with them full time had added even more pressure. Janet also expressed annoyance with telephone calls from Kinesha's mother, which seemed to have gotten more frequent since the couple's marriage.

Robert said that things did not seem so hard to him. He was finishing his last semester to complete his bachelor's degree and was working part time. He thought that Janet was impatient with Kinesha because Janet did not like Kinesha's mother. Janet shook her head as Robert spoke. I asked about how the children were adjusting to all the changes—their parents' marriage, the move to a new home, changing schools, and acquiring new sibling(s). Again, Janet spoke first. She said that her boys were doing fine but that Kinesha was a lot of trouble. She did not follow instructions, was often disrespectful, did not pick up after herself, told lies, and did not know how to keep herself clean. When Kinesha spent the weekend at their house, Kinesha's mother called too many times, and from Janet's perspective, the only purpose of these calls was to upset everyone. She said that Kinesha was too clingy with Robert and that she was too old to act like that.

Robert said that he agreed with Janet's opinion that Kinesha's mother is a difficult woman, which was exactly why he wanted Kinesha to live with them. He said he wanted Kinesha to have a woman like Janet as an example, and he wanted Janet to help him to do for Kinesha what he was helping her do for her boys. At the end of the first session, I told the couple that I would be happy to work with them. I identified several of their strengths, including how much each of them wanted to provide a good family for their children. Although I believed that the couple was struggling with many stressors beyond Kinesha's behavior, I felt that my credibility with this couple and their commitment to therapy were dependent on my attention and skill in addressing their issues of concern about Kinesha.

I explained how the managed care company worked and how information about our work together would be shared with the insurance company. I explained my policy to communicate with the managed care company only in writing and to submit diagnostic assessments, treatment plans, and reports only after providing patients with an opportunity to review them.

I said I appreciated how difficult it was to talk to a complete stranger about their personal business. I told them that if they wanted to schedule another appointment, we could do that now. If they preferred to take some time to decide about whether they wanted to come back, they could take a few days to think about it and talk with each other, giving me a call if they wanted to meet again. I have found that giving clients the choice about scheduling a next appointment lets them know they have the right to decide whether or not they want to come back and gives them a graceful way to exit if they choose not to return. The Smith family opted to return.

I worked with this family using a combination of individual sessions with each parent, sessions with the couple, sessions with the entire family, and sessions with Kinesha and Robert and Kinesha and Janet. As noted, we met for a total of 18 sessions over the course of 7 months. I chose not to see Kinesha in individual sessions because I anticipated a relatively short-term course of treatment, due to limits on the number of sessions imposed by the family's insurance benefits. In my judgment, the most efficient use of the time available to us would involve a focus on strengthening the relationships of parent–child and husband–wife. In our first session I suggested this approach for Janet's and Robert's consideration, and they agreed.

We established the following goals for our work:

1. Strengthen the connection between Janet and Kinesha.
2. Help Kinesha adjust to new home, new family members, and new school.
3. Help Janet and Robert establish their new family identity and support the children in honoring and maintaining positive relationships with their noncustodial parents.
4. Help the family develop strategies for maintaining respectful connection during moments of conflict and disagreement.

Building Connections

In our first few sessions I helped Janet and Robert identify some steps they could take immediately to establish themselves as a new family—activities they could do together, division of labor to accomplish household chores, and house rules they could establish. I suggested that we begin our work together by practicing on the smaller problems. I was hoping that their trust in me and a sense of value for our work together would develop through experiences of success in the accomplishment of concrete tasks. I asked for permission to contact Kinesha's school so that I could talk to her teacher about school performance and to find out what counseling or other services might be available to her at her school. Shortly after our work began, Kinesha moved into the Smith home, and Kinesha's mother, Kim, moved to a new community a considerable distance away.

I encouraged Robert to meet with Kinesha's teachers, and he agreed. I believed that Robert's action in relationship on Kinesha's behalf had great potential for deepening the connection between Robert and Kinesha, between Robert and Janet, and between Janet and Kinesha. His willingness also helped to enhance his identity as a competent, capable husband and father. The attention from her father and his participation in her school showed Kinesha that she was special and important to him. Robert's efforts with Kinesha's school resulted in her participation in several special academic and social programs. Robert and Kinesha bonded around their similar school struggles, and Robert encouraged and praised Kinesha's progress and accomplishments. Janet was pleased with the positive changes in Kinesha's behavior and appearance. Kinesha became less clingy, as she became more secure in her relationship with her father. Janet felt supported by Robert's willingness to take responsibility for Kinesha and appreciated the care he provided for her sons. At the same time, Janet became less threatened by, and more understanding and supportive of, Kinesha's need to maintain a relationship with her mother while establishing and negotiating her own important but different role in Kenisha's life. Robert felt competent, capable, and successful in his roles as both husband and father. Things in the family were getting better.

In one of our early couple sessions, Janet asked me about how I worked, what theories I used, and how I thought therapy would help. Often clients ask for reading materials that describe relational–cultural theory, or they ask for direction to articles or books that could be helpful to them in exploring whatever issues they are dealing with in therapy. In managed care cases where treatment is time limited, I encourage supplementing our work with reading materials, especially when the clients request them. Janet asked for relational–cultural reading materials about remarried families, raising stepchildren, and challenges faced by women in the workplace. Among the materials I gave her was Clevonne Turner's 1984 article, "Psychosocial Barriers to Black Women's Career Development." After reading the article, Janet described her own "learned talents to survive" and her view of herself as capable and, in some ways, obligated to pass on these talents to Kenisha. Janet was also able to frame some of Kenisha's troubling behaviors as strategies of disconnection—ways that Kenisha behaved to protect herself from being hurt when she anticipated being ignored or rejected. Janet was able to replace anger toward Kenisha with empathy, as she understood that Kenisha's behaviors were expressions of her fears of being ignored, abandoned, and hurt. Janet was able to help Kenisha see herself as strong, smart, responsible, and lovable. In response, Kenisha began to behave differently.

I also gave Robert and Janet a copy of "The Five Good Things"

(Miller, 1988), which describes the qualities of a growth-producing relationship:

1. A sense of zest or energy that comes from connecting with another person(s).
2. The ability and motivation to take action in the relationships as well as in other situations.
3. An increased knowledge of oneself and the other person(s).
4. An increased sense of worth.
5. A desire for more connections beyond the particular one.

I expanded on the points by giving examples that illustrated how each of the five points would look in family relationships. I expressed hope that our work together would help them strengthen their relationships to each other. To emphasize how much I valued The Five Good Things, I humorously told them that I kept a copy of The Five Good Things right next to a copy of the Ten Commandments. Janet and Robert talked about their wish to create a growth-producing home for everyone in their family. I thought about the importance of creating a sense of safety and the value of supportive family relationships for all children but especially for children of color, where home and family can be a refuge from the harshness and cruelty of a racist world. At a subsequent family session, Kinesha carried in a poster the family had created: The poster, which was labeled "Smith Family—Five Good People," was a collage that had a picture of each family member and pictures of each person's special gifts. Janet said that the poster was displayed on the refrigerator next to a copy of the Ten Commandments—something that was common to both the Catholic and Baptist religions that were part of this new blended family. I was moved by the family's greater connection to each other and their desire to show me how something I had offered them had been re-created in such a personal and unique way. This was a moment of mutual empathy. Jordan (1997) describes mutual empathy as occurring when the client knows, sees, and recognizes that the therapist is moved, touched, and affected by his or her experience. I felt a greater connection to the family and a greater investment in our work. The family's acceptance of what I had offered them and their reframing of The Five Good Things as Five Good People provided all of us with a relational experience of contributing something valuable that led to further creativity through relationship.

Racial Images as Threats to Connection

Our work together presented us with several opportunities to stretch our capacity to speak with authenticity about race. Many of the relational images of white people held by members of this family were of people who judged them, disrespected them, dismissed them, and treated them badly in a painful variety of ways. One week, Robert reported that he had gotten a poor grade on an exam and that when he went to talk to the professor, he felt dismissed. In discussing what happened, I learned that Robert had gone to the professor's office just as the professor had been getting ready to leave. The professor told Robert that he would need to come back during his office hours later in the week. Robert explained that he worked a part-time job and would not be able to meet during the professor's office hours. The professor said he was sorry that his office hours were not convenient and hoped Robert would be able to work something out. Robert expressed the wish to drop the course so that he would not have to continue to interact with the professor. He was considering taking the course the following semester, even though that would delay his graduation. He described the professor, a white man, as arrogant, rude, and rigid. I empathized with Robert's experience of being treated rudely. Robert's school had a reputation for being hard on its students. I wondered aloud what part racism played in the disconnection between Robert and the professor and whether exploring that with Robert would be helpful. Robert observed that our talking about the professor's motives was not going to change the outcome. I thought about my own experiences in college with difficult professors but chose to keep the observations of similar experiences to myself. That week we discussed Robert's options for dealing with this professor and finishing the course.

Another week Janet described being upset with a coworker who had scheduled an important client presentation on a day when Janet had planned to be on vacation. The coworker was a white woman with whom Janet had what she described as a cooperative but distant relationship. As she told me the story, I was reminded of a similar experience I had had years ago. While I was on vacation, my supervisor scheduled an important meeting about funding for a project that I had been managing. When I asked him about scheduling the meeting when he did, he said that it simply had not occurred to him that it would have been important to me to schedule the meeting when I could be there. I did not share the memory of my experience with Janet, but held the memory and the feelings it engendered in my mind as Janet and I discussed how she might address the issue with her coworker.

At another session, we discussed James's new refusal to attend school. He had stayed home for several days, complaining of a variety of vague physical ailments. On the day Janet insisted that he return to school, she received a call at work from the school asking why James was not in class. Janet panicked. When she could not reach Robert, she rushed home to find James watching television and eating ice cream. We discovered that

James's beloved teacher was on sick leave and had been replaced by a new "mean" teacher. The new mean teacher was a white woman.

When I listened to the family members tell those stories, I felt as if our relationship was at risk. In each of those incidents I felt angry and sad for my clients and the tangle of social forces they faced daily. I also felt constricted by the grip of shame, the "white guilt," afraid that my clients would see me as "one of them." I struggled to find the courage to name racism as the source of pain in each of these interactions and expressed my genuine desire to find respectful words to initiate an exploration of its destructive power. I wondered aloud with them if raising the question of racism would increase rather than reduce their pain? I did not know if my clients' reluctance to name racism as an issue in the interactions described above was simply avoidance of a difficult topic or evidence of their belief that they did not think that I, as a white person, would "get it" if they did. I acknowledged that sometimes I did not get it. Sometimes I felt that my clients had so many relational images of untrustworthy white people that it was too much to overcome; there were too many negative experiences in their histories to trust me enough to risk being authentic. And I had a lifetime of my own negative relational images of blacks to recognize and confront: the difficult, unfair black professor from my past, the black secretary who accused me of racism because I complained about poor work performance, the uneasy feeling I would get when a black man and I stood alone in an elevator or at a bus stop at night, not to mention all the myths, beliefs, and stereotypes of "those people" that had the power to influence how I thought, felt, and behaved in a relationship with a person of color. The grip of shame has the power to choke relational possibility, to render us empty and speechless. It is only through our courage to risk and our capacity to acknowledge both our yearnings for connection and our fears that the grip can be loosened enough to create the potential for a healing connection.

Examining Disconnections

Information about the couple's large extended family identified several family members who were sources of strength and support for the couple. Robert's uncle helped with tuition expenses and provided Robert with a well-paying part-time job that accommodated his school schedule. Janet's parents and her sister were willing to provide child care when needed. Janet's cousins had helped the family get a mortgage to purchase their new home, and Robert's brothers had helped with home repair and painting. Longstanding relationships among all these relatives had been changed by the creation of the newly blended Smith family. Janet came from a college-educated, Midwestern urban family, and Robert came from a Southern rural background. He was the first in his family to attend college. Janet's family was Roman Catholic, and Robert's family was Baptist. The couple had some disagreements about which religion would have a place in their life. Both sides of the extended family had been disappointed when Robert and Janet had decided to be married in a civil ceremony. Janet and Robert were clear that they did not want more children, but Janet had been troubled by questions from relatives about when Janet and Robert would be having a baby. Janet's family had been outwardly supportive of her marriage to Robert, but she believed that some members of her family believed she was "marrying down." When Janet first introduced Robert to her younger sister, her sister had made the comment that she hoped Janet was not settling for Robert because she was panicked about the shortage of "quality" black men. Janet felt hurt by her sister's comment but never discussed it with her. Janet noticed that whenever they were with her sister, she (Janet) became annoyed with Robert's "country ways" and critical of his clothing and imperfect grammar.

Both Robert and Janet were struggling to negotiate their place as parent to each other's children and to reconcile the parenting roles, responsibilities, and relationships with each of their former partners. Janet's former partner was inconsistent in his contact with their sons. He was unable to maintain employment and was not able to provide any financial support. Robert had little competition in his role as father to Janet's boys. It seemed that the boys welcomed him, and Robert and the boys enjoyed having each other as part of their respective lives. Kinesha apparently felt strong loyalty conflicts in her efforts to form a relationship with her new stepmother. Janet identified some significant differences between herself and Kinesha's mother, Kim. Janet described Kim as a large, sloppy woman. She said that Kim never had clean clothes for Kinesha and had not taught Kinesha anything about how to behave or how to take care of herself. Janet said that Kim had not been able to mother Kinesha since she was born, that Kinesha was always sent from house to house, and that Robert's mother spoiled Kinesha because she felt sorry for that the child had "such a horrible mother." Janet said she was embarrassed to take Kinesha anywhere because of how she looked and how she behaved. Furthermore, Janet's efforts to help Kinesha with grooming or clothing selection were often met with resistance by Kinesha.

Janet was often harsh and critical, and sometimes even unkind, in her descriptions of Kinesha and Kim. Janet often presented Kinesha with choices that required Kinesha to choose between Mother's ways and Stepmother's ways. Janet would describe conversations with Kinesha wherein Janet had intended to express words of encouragement to Kinesha but which, to Kinesha, sounded critical of Kim. I saw the struggle of competition that is frequently part of the relationship between stepparent and stepchild in remarried families. I tried to help Janet see that Kinesha's rejection of Janet's attempts to influence her in grooming, behavior, and dress were more a reflection of Kinesha's loyalty to Kim than of her rejection of Janet or disrespect of Janet's authority. I wanted to help Janet see how much Kinesha needed *both* her mother *and* Janet. I struggled to find a way to praise Janet's efforts with Kinesha and to empathize with Janet's disappointment when Kenisha responded negatively to Janet's attempts at mothering. In one session I shared an observation that it was probably difficult for someone like Janet to understand how Kim could take such poor care of her daughter. I said I noticed how much thought, effort, and time Janet put into the care of her children. Janet's eyes filled with tears, as she spoke about how hard she tried with Kinesha, but that she was afraid that she could not help Kinesha, because Kinesha was just too much like Kim.

Janet also talked about her feelings regarding the physical differences between herself and Kinesha—Kinesha's large size, dark skin, and "bad" hair. Trotman (2000) notes that the physical characteristics that distinguish African American women, such as skin color, hair texture, facial features, and body type, can be the basis of adverse treatment by family members and by the greater African American community. Our relationship gave Janet a place to express her difficulty in being loving and motherly toward Kinesha, when Kinesha looked nothing like the daughter she would have wanted. Janet's image of her stepmother role was one of someone who loved her stepchild as her own; her idealized image of stepdaughter was of someone who wanted to be like her and who would appreciate and accept her expressions of care. We talked about how operating under the tyranny of these idealized and unrealistic relational images (D. Littlefield, personal communication, 1999) prevented Janet and Kinesha from being themselves with each other. We compared the image of stepmother to the relational image of "othermother" (Collins, 1987)—that is, a woman who supports children whose biological mothers are ill-prepared or unable to care for them. The relational image of "othermother" offered greater possibility and enabled Janet to be more generous and empathic with Kinesha's struggles with loyalty conflicts and to the disappointments Kinesha experienced in her relationship with her mother.

Disconnection and Repair through Difference

In one of the couple sessions, Janet and Robert told me about an incident of disagreement over the use of physical punishment as a method of disciplining their children. Janet believed that physical punishment ("spanking," not beating) was sometimes the only way to get the children to listen. Robert disagreed with that practice and had expressed his disagreement in front of the children. Janet believed that Robert had undermined her authority. Instead of attending to Janet's and Robert's feelings and the disconnection between the two of them, I tried to lead them to explore other effective techniques of disciplining the children. Janet became quite agitated, commenting, "Well, I'm not surprised that you're siding with him." When I asked her why she thought I was "siding" with Robert, she said, "White people let their children disrespect their parents [adding under her breath] and everyone else, and they don't do anything about it." I felt hurt by her comment and heard in it a message that she had felt disrespected by me. I, in turn, felt challenged and disrespected by Janet. I was tempted to disconnect to protect my feelings and hide my vulnerability behind a mask of professional power, detachment, and psuedo-objectivity. I could respond with "professional defensiveness." I tried to go back to Janet's feelings of being undermined by Robert, but I could not figure out a way to be empathic to Janet, Robert, and the children, *and* respond authentically at the same time. I said something like, "I can imagine how sometimes hitting the children may seem like the only thing to do to get them to obey." Janet looked at me and said, "Well, what exactly do you do when your children disobey?" I stopped for a moment and thought, "now what?" I had no children. Do I answer the question or explore what is underneath it? I think that, generally, when clients ask personal questions of their therapists, they are asking for confirmation that the therapist can understand them and their circumstances. I think they are asking: "How are you like me? What life experience do you have that will enable you to help me? Can you understand me?" By probing for examples that demonstrate ways in which the therapist has faced similar challenges, the client is looking for evidence of the likelihood of empathy and understanding and what Trotman (2000) describes as a "deeper experience of kinship" (p. 263). This was not the first time my own parenting practices have been questioned by clients. On this issue of disclosure, Janet Surrey (Miller, Jordan, Kaplan, Stiver, & Surrey, 1991) notes:

> When I think about the criteria I use to decide about verbal or conscious disclosure, they center around the potential impact on the client, myself, and the relationship. Will this help move the relationship toward expanded connection? Will it enhance the possibilities of empathic joining, either through my reaching out to join the client or, sometimes, by asking the client to stretch to encompass something difficult to hear from me? (p. 11)

As I quickly ran though my lexicon of possible responses, only an honest answer to the question seemed like the right thing to say. I also considered that my credibility as a family therapist might suffer when I told

Janet and Robert that I was not a parent. I believed that Janet was simultaneously asking for some specific information and telling me that she felt
hurt and disconnected by Robert's criticism and by my failure to "get"
how she had been hurt. I said, "Janet, I can tell you that I don't think physical punishment is effective in disciplining children. I don't believe in it. I
think it's wrong. And [I said this part more loudly] I am *not* a mother. Being a mother is a very hard job, and I don't know what I might do if I had
the job of raising children—trying to teach them, protect them, and keep
them safe." I was trying to honestly express my position on physical punishment and humbly acknowledge that my position had never been put to
the test by the real-life challenges of being a parent.

Robert took the moment to apologize to Janet for not supporting her
in front of the children. He praised her skills as a mother. Robert said that
his own father believed in hitting, and as a result, he had spent a lot of
years being both afraid and angry. He did not want his children to grow
up being afraid and angry. Robert described the harsh beatings he had
suffered at his father's hands. Janet also had been hit as a child, and she
believed that she and her siblings had become (perhaps, as a result of
physical punishment) good people who "knew the difference between
right and wrong."

Janet looked at me and said, "I'll bet you never got hit." Again I
paused and thought about how to respond. I allowed my own childhood
memories of being hurt, frightened, and confused to run through my
mind as I thought about how I could respond authentically from my function as therapist in a way that would contribute to a forward movement in
my relationship with this family. I told Janet and Robert that I did get hit
as a child. I explained that my parents learned that way of discipline from
their parents, and I think they did it because they did not know what else
to do. They wanted me to learn right from wrong, and they thought it
would stop me from doing things they did not want me to do. I told them
that while it was likely that sometimes the threat or memory of getting hit
stopped me from disobeying, I also remembered the hurt long after the
experience—not only the physical hurt but the hurt in my heart and spirit
too. I expressed my belief that hitting may have stopped me from doing
wrong, but that one person hitting another was not likely to create a
growth-producing relationship for either the person being hit or the person doing the hitting. As Janet and Robert left the session, I encouraged
them to keep talking about how they would discipline the children in a
way that would be "growth producing," how they could support each
other's authority, and how they would handle disagreements like this in
the future.

This was an important juncture in our work together, and one
wherein I was presented with an opportunity to face and transform a pro-

fessional strategy of disconnection. When I felt challenged and disrespected by Janet, I was tempted to use a "power-over" strategy by protecting my feelings and hiding my vulnerability behind a mask of professional detachment and objectivity and responding with professional defensiveness. Instead, by listening to Janet and Robert and being empathic with myself, my parents, my own feelings of both competence and inadequacy as a person and a therapist, and simultaneously with Janet's and Robert's desires to be good parents to their children, I was able to transform a potential power-over moment (i.e., responding with defensiveness and reactivity) with what Jordan (1995) describes as a more relational "power with"—responding with a sense of responsibility for the care of the relationship and a sensitivity to the history of warmth and mutual positive regard that were part of our connection.

Building Strategies to Maintain Connection

An important part of the work with this family involved helping them stay in connection to their commitment to each other during conflict and to increase their capacity to see anger and conflict as a resource to improve their connection (Miller & Surrey, 1997). We worked together at observing and understanding their relational patterns of movement from connection to disconnection and developed and practiced respectful strategies for staying connected in conflict and for reconnection. Janet's and Robert's relational strategies of disconnection toward each other often resulted in each responding with further strategies of disconnection. Robert's typical strategies were to withdraw and express less of his authentic self, whereas Janet's were to become loud, demanding, critical, and impatient. When each partner was able to identify his or her strategies of disconnection and see how those strategies blocked each one's capacity for mutual empathy, each was more willing to identify his or her own part in the disconnection and change in behavior toward one another without blaming the other or feeling like he or she was giving up important parts of him- or herself. Over the course of the work, the couple developed what we called "strategies of caring connection"—mutual empathy for the self, the other, and the relationship. These strategies included (1) *speaking softly, slowly, and with sense of good timing* in raising concerns and expressing complaints. This mode of communication promotes a spirit of calm and openness of head and heart in both speaker and listener, as opposed to shouting complaints as the other is involved in another activity. (2) *Giving the other time to take it in*, after offering an opinion, preference, or suggestion, allows the other person time to consider the wishes of the speaker and to respond without feeling controlled, overruled, or pressured. (3) *Giving credit and leading with gratitude* expressing thanks, gratitude, and appreciation to the other for acts of generosity, accommodation, consideration, thoughtfulness, and kindness.

The couple identified many differences in beliefs about such things as child discipline, religion, relationships with extended family, and saving and spending money. Helping the couple negotiate these differences and develop strategies to respectfully discuss conflict while staying connected to their commitment to each other was the foundation of our work. Another important piece of the work was to reinforce the strengths of each parent and helping each to see that the differences between them as individuals were a benefit to them as a couple. When Janet saw Robert as being too slow in getting things done, too easy on the children, and not firm enough in enforcing rules, we identified Robert's patience and ability to get the children to do homework and household tasks by making things a game. When Robert saw Janet as rigid, bossy, and too concerned with how everything and everybody looks, we identified Janet's ability to accomplish a million things at once, select clothing that helped everybody look their best, and create a comfortable home that had "a place for everything and everything in its place."

The Smith family and I worked hard at being authentic. We courageously and imperfectly confronted issues of race, power, and conflict. I was moved by their efforts to connect with each other and with me and by how hard they were willing to work at creating a home and a future for their new family.

After 7 months, we ended our work together, pleased with what we had accomplished. Robert had passed the course with the difficult professor and completed his degree. Janet's support in his job search resulted in his being the first of his graduating class to be employed. Janet's sister gave a toast at Robert's graduation party, praising him and expressing pride that he was part of her family. The relationship between Janet and Kinesha had become less conflicted. Kinesha was becoming a loving older sister to her two younger brothers, doing better in school, and excelling in art classes. When Kinesha graduated from middle school, Robert and Janet supported Kinesha's need for a relationship with her mother by inviting Kim to attend Kinesha's graduation. Janet framed several family photographs for Kinesha's room, including one of Kinesha and Janet together and one of Kinesha and Kim. Janet and Robert said they felt closer to each other and more supported by each other. Before Robert started his new job, he surprised Janet by arranging a weekend trip for just the two of them without the children.

The Smith family left our work with a deepened sense of their connection to each other as a family and a greater ability to manage and understand the inevitable flow of connection and disconnection that are part of all relationships. They developed loving, respectful, and authentic strategies for reconnection that would help to keep them united when difficulty with their differences and conflict among them threatened their connections to each other. I thank them for giving me the opportunity to share the story of our healing connection.

REFERENCES

Boyd-Franklin, N. (2003). *Black families in therapy: Understanding the African American experience* (2nd ed.). New York: Guilford Press.

Collins, P. H. (1987). The meaning of motherhood in black culture. *Sage: A Scholarly Journal on Black Women, 4*, 3–10.

Gwyn, F., & Kilpatrick, A. (1981). Family therapy with low-income blacks: A tool or turn-off? *Social Casework, 62*, 259–266.

Jenkins, Y. M. (2000). The Stone Center theoretical approach revisited: Applications for African American women. In L. C. Jackson & B. Greene (Eds.), *Psychotherapy with African American women: Innovations in psychodynamic perspectives and practice* (pp. 62–81). New York: Guilford Press.

Jordan, J. V. (1991). Empathy, mutuality, and therapeutic change: Clinical implications of a relational model. In J. V. Jordan, A. G. Kaplan, J. B. Miller, I. P. Stiver, & J. L. Surrey (Eds.), *Women's growth in connection: Writings from the Stone Center* (pp. 283–290). New York: Guilford Press.

Jordan, J. V. (1995). Relational awareness: Transforming disconnection. *Work in Progress, No. 76*. Wellesley, MA: Stone Center Working Paper Series.

Jordan, J. V. (1997). A relational perspective for understanding women's development. In J. V. Jordan (Ed.), *Women's growth in diversity: More writings from the Stone Center* (pp. 9–24). New York: Guilford Press.

Miller, J. B. (1988). Connections, disconnections, and violations. *Work in Progress, No. 33*. Wellesley, MA: Stone Center Working Paper Series.

Miller, J. B., Jordan, J. V., Kaplan, A., Stiver, I. P., & Surrey, J. L. (1991). Some misconceptions and reconceptions of a relational approach. *Work in Progess, No. 49*. Wellesley, MA: Stone Center Working Paper Series.

Miller, J. B., & Stiver, L. (1998). *The healing connection: How women form relationships in therapy and in life*. Boston: Beacon Press.

Miller, J. B., & Surrey, J. (1997). Rethinking women's anger: The personal and the global. In J. V. Jordan (Ed.), *Women's growth in diversity: More writings from the Stone Center* (pp. 199–216). New York: Guilford Press.

Steinhorn, L., & Diggs-Brown, B. (1999). *By the color of our skin: The illusion of integration and the reality of race*. New York: Dutton/Penguin.

Sue, S. (1977). Community mental health services to minority groups: Some optimism, some pessimism. *American Psychologist, 32*, 616–624.

Sue, S., McKinney, H., Allen, D., & Hall, J. (1974). Delivery of community mental health services to black and white clients. *Journal of Consulting and Clinical Psychology, 42*, 794–801.

Trotman, F. K. (2000). Feminist psychodynamic psychotherapy with African American women: Some differences. In L. C. Jackson & B. Greene (Eds.), *Psychothera-py with African American women: Innovations in psychodynamic perspectives and practice* (pp. 251–274). New York: Guilford Press.

Turner, C. (1984). Psychosocial barriers to black women's career development. *Work in Progress, No. 15*. Wellesley, MA: Stone Center Working Paper Series.

Walker, M. (1999). Race, self, and society: Relational challenges in a culture of dis-connection. *Work in Progress, No. 85*. Wellesley, MA: Stone Center Working Paper Series.

10

Relational Movement in Group Psychotherapy

Nikki Fedele

RELATIONAL–CULTURAL THEORY AND GROUP PSYCHOTHERAPY

Relationships are the essential elements of a group therapy experience. Although most group therapists would agree that relationships are critical to healing in groups, a relational–cultural group therapy model emphasizes movement from disconnection to stronger, deeper connection as the critical factor. This is true of the "here-and-now" group interactions as well as the replay of past "there-and-then" relationships in a group. Initially, members do not feel safe enough to fully represent themselves in their group encounters. Although disconnections in relationships are inevitable, members are urged to engage in empathic discussion about their disconnections. Participants begin to identify the disavowed parts of themselves and examine patterns of their interactions in the group. They discover the strategies of disconnection and the relational images (Miller & Stiver, 1995, 1997) that underlie their behavior and use the group as a laboratory to unravel and understand the emotional roots of these strongholds of dysfunctional behavior. The experience of mutual empathy in this relational space allows members to examine and modify relational images rooted in the past and replayed in the present (Fedele, 2001). Furthermore, they begin to understand the strong cultural controlling images that play a formative role in their development (Collins, 2000; Jordan, Walker, & Miller, 2001). A relational–cultural understanding of group dynamics provides a context for understanding change and healing in group psychotherapy.

THE GROUP CONTEXT

The context of this case is a group whose members were all women in the age range of 30–55 years. The group, although homogeneous around gender and race, was heterogeneous in terms of class, sexual orientation, marital status, and parenthood. Membership in the group changed over the course of the 4 years that the relationship developed between two members, who are called "Audrey" and "Carla." The demographic data, although essentially giving an accurate impression, has been disguised; the actual clinical material is a composite from a number of group interactions. For the purposes of this chapter, the clinical focus is on these two members in the group, their strategies of disconnection, their relational images, how they engaged with each other, with the leader and other members, and how their relational images interlocked in the group. The presentation includes the resolution of some moments of impasse.

An Introduction to Audrey

Audrey was a 45-year-old married mother of two teenagers who lived in an affluent suburb. She was from a well-to-do Italian family, strongly identified with the Italian culture, yet she had married a highly successful man outside her Catholic faith. Although she had struggled with a debilitating bipolar depression, she had owned her own successful fine art gallery for many years. At the first individual interview for the group, she presented in an overall engaging way. However, Audrey's perfect appearance and slightly pressured, anxious quality was quite apparent. I was somewhat put off by Audrey's primary concern that the group members might be too depressed for her. I asked for clarification, and she explained by relating her previous experience with another group leader. That therapist had assured Audrey, in the initial individual interviews, that that group for depressed women would be suitable for her. During the first session of this previous group, Audrey was overwhelmed by intense anxiety because she perceived the members as severely depressed and unable to interact. She never returned to that group and felt tricked by the therapist. In the course of our interview, Audrey suggested that she come to one group session to try it out. Such a procedure, of course, would be devastating to the current group's members who would feel as if they had not made the grade.

My initial impression was that Audrey desperately wanted to be in a group, but that it had to be the perfect one. If it was perfect, then it could contain and possibly overshadow her imperfections. Audrey was frightened of acknowledging her depression and the deep disappointment and sadness it caused her. Her relational image involved a deep-rooted sense of not being good enough. Audrey's strategies of disconnection included the questions (1) "Is this group good enough for me?" and (2) "Is this therapist good enough for me?" Her presentation activated many of my own relational images around being good enough and the wish to be the perfect therapist or even, more soberly, the good-enough therapist. I was able to actively keep my own strategies of disconnection in check, probably due to her likeable and engaging presentation. The distancing strategies that I could have acted on were anger at her presumption and questioning of my abilities, as well as discomfort with her meticulous and impeccably fashionable appearance. My strategies of disconnection might have caused me to confront her strategies or question her commitment to joining a group.

On the contrary, I struggled to find the empathic response that respected and addressed Audrey's paradox. It was important to empathize with her wish to be understood and feel as if she belonged at the same time that her feelings about the group were validated. I acknowledged that, as the group therapist, I could make a mistake in adding her to the group, but that my best sense was that the match would, in fact, work. I recognized her request as understandable but explained the important reasons for the usual 3-month commitment. Audrey decided to trust my conviction that the group would be a good match for her needs. Her ability to move toward the group while acknowledging her fears demonstrates the emotional movement that an empathic and empowering therapeutic stance can generate. Empathizing with the strategy of disconnection, while acknowledging the paradoxical need to belong, is an integral facet of a relational–cultural approach to both individual and group treatment.

Audrey presented with extreme anxiety about her mental handicap. Because of the debilitating nature of her previous depressive episodes, she was terrified that joining a group would somehow precipitate a new bout of depression. At the same time, she experienced deep pain about her loneliness and cried openly, at the pregroup interview, about her inability to talk about these feelings with anyone. Clearly, she yearned to share her intense feelings, but she had developed a strategy of disconnection that involved avoiding those feelings. She disconnected from both her own feelings as well as her ability to connect with others around those feelings. Since this dual disconnection interfered with her capacity to resolve these issues and grow from her experiences, she was stuck and unable to move forward. Audrey's behavior appeared to be aimed at avoiding difficult feelings in the group—both her own and other members'. She was frightened to face her feelings of inadequacy and limitation. But her strategies of disconnection, though ostensibly protecting her, also caused her to feel isolated and alone. This paradox was a major theme for Audrey's subsequent work in the group.

An Introduction to Carla

Carla was a married woman of about 50 years who had two children in their early teens. She had been raised in the South in a poor white Protestant family that included a sister and a brother. Her initial presentation was rather austere, and she appeared worn and tired. She seemed to pay little attention to her appearance and looked older than her stated age. Carla expressed a strong religious belief that fueled her commitment to a life of caretaking. She had recently moved with her husband and two children to New England. She was employed at a position in mental health that, although quite demanding, was only minimally compensated. At the same time she was trying to pursue advanced studies in her field. During the course of the group, she had increasing financial concerns because her husband lost his employment.

Carla sought a group therapeutic experience because of her anger. A supervisor at her work/studies program had insisted that she attend group therapy, because she exhibited disruptive anger in her interactions. In fact, they had offered to pay for the sessions. Her initial presentation in the pregroup interview suggested that she was extremely committed and sincere in her efforts to deal with this problem. She openly discussed her anger as a problem that needed work; however, at her first group meeting, she directed a great deal of anger toward her supervisors in a harsh, provocative manner. This was a disconnecting presentation for an initial meeting. As the leader, I was surprised by the intensity of the feelings she expressed, and I was concerned that she, being angry with me as the authority figure, would disrupt the group. The members expressed their fears that Carla would become enraged in the group, that they might not be able to handle it, and that her presence could disconnect them all. This possibility activated, in members and myself, relational images from the past in which anger is perceived as destructive in relationships, or, alternately, that a person cannot be loved or be loving if he or she is angry. Carla's anger was an effective strategy of disconnection, since it distanced her from others and caused her to attempt to be disconnected from her feelings.

I was struck by the contrast between my initial impression of Carla during the pregroup interview and her presentation in the more stressful group format. Something about being in a group for the first time caused her to appear stern and unrelenting. In the individual interview, I recalled my perception of Carla's sincerity, her search for connection, and the sadness that lived beneath her anger. I expressed this dilemma by empathizing with the difficulty of joining a group as a new member, but wondered why Carla expressed such intense anger in her first meeting. I shared my concern about the disconnection that her anger and the group's fears could induce. Carla responded well to my curiosity about her off-putting behavior. She was able to examine her anxiety about beginning the group, and she could talk about trying to protect herself from criticism. Her willingness and honesty caused a shift in the dynamics of the group. Members began to empathize with Carla's experience. She could then express hurt about the criticism of her supervisors and about the tremendous sadness that she felt because of her anger. Bearing so much anger was a terrible burden. Carla's goal was apparent: She needed to understand the roots of this anger and her inability to connect with her feelings of sadness and inadequacy. The opportunity afforded by Carla's admission to the group was also evident: We would, no doubt, be called upon to identify and examine our own relational images and strategies of disconnection concerning anger and vulnerability.

Carla was hoping to improve her relationships with her friends, her coworkers, and her family. She was thrilled that her employing organization was footing the bill. She remained in the group for about 2 years and reported back, from time to time, that her supervisors felt that she was making progress. Carla experienced the support of her organization as extremely caring, even in the face of her anger and hurt. She would often talk about her Southern background as a way to distinguish her Protestant heritage from what she perceived as a more constrained New England one. She was also very conscious of class issues and of her lower-class background, at one point referring to her family's social status as "white trash." Carla had difficulty with what she perceived as the more Puritanical and inauthentic reserve of many of her colleagues and acquaintances. She experienced them as extremely judgmental and not forthcoming, but was able to examine these perceptions and their underlying assumptions in the group. Her fears of judgment could be addressed because they were rooted both in the relational images stemming from her relationship to her mother and from class issues.

At one point, Carla tearfully related her experience at her mother's bedside during an illness. She experienced her mother as critical and unwavering even then and described sadness and rage over her wishes to please her mother. The relational paradox involved Carla's yearning for her mother's approval, on the one hand, at the same time that she was furious that this approval was unattainable, on the other. Her disconnections seemed to intensify around the shame and guilt she experienced when she felt the full force of her anger at her psychologically abusive mother. Shame and guilt also seemed to be interwoven with her feelings about social class. The relational images were "I am not good enough for my mother to love me" and "I am not good enough because of my poverty," and her strategies of disconnection included the anger, shame, and guilt that derailed her relationships. These images and strategies were elucidated during the initial course of the group and formed the basis of later group interventions.

THE MAJOR RELATIONAL THEMES

The therapeutic work in groups involves unraveling the history of each member's experiences and the elaborations of those experiences. The initial effort of group therapy involves teaching members to notice when they feel connected or disconnected and how to get reconnected. The members of this particular group developed what they called the mantra of the group: *"Talk about disconnection in the group, and you will feel connected."* The next step involves the elaboration of the strategies of disconnection, which become obvious via interactions in the group. The leader and members begin to identify patterns in strategies of disconnection for each member and look to see the ways they interlock.

Audrey had grown up in an upper-middle-class home with a mother she experienced as critical and a father who adored his oldest daughter. She had a reasonably normal relationship with her younger sister, characterized by both competition and warmth. She experienced herself as the pretty one, as opposed to her sister, the smart one. The pivotal experience for Audrey was the untimely death of her father, a very successful businessman, of a massive, fatal cardiac arrest when she turned 20. At that time, her family's financial security was threatened because of his sudden death, and Audrey experienced pressure to marry someone who could take care of her. Audrey's relationship with her mother had been conflicted prior to her father's death, but his loss strained the relationship even further. Her mother had always set high standards of behavior and appearance that did not allow for demonstrations of sadness, vulnerability, or incapacity. In order to avoid criticism, Audrey attempted to meet these standards by developing a competent, caretaking role in the family as the older sister, particularly after her father's death. Her relational images around her relationship with her mother included "I am not good enough for people to love me." Since a number of other members experienced the loss of loved ones during her time in the group, Audrey felt comfortable expressing her sadness in the group around the unresolved loss of her father on a number of occasions. She was able to share in the group her wishes that he were alive, so she could seek his approval of her career, her children, her house, and her husband's success. Audrey brought to the group a set of relational images that reflected her experience in these compromised family relationships.

Audrey had constructed a self-disparaging view of herself when she could not engage with anyone in her family around her fears or her anxiety. The pressure to look good and overcome adversity did not leave room for these difficult feelings. Audrey, believing that caretaking was her primary avenue to relationship in her family, developed into an adult caretaker who had difficulty allowing herself any feelings or experiences that contradicted that role. Her vulnerability to depression exacerbated her fear of feeling inadequate and of losing the regard of others. Although being a caretaker certainly was a positive role for her, at times it had also become a strategy for disconnection with her children, because it allowed her to disconnect from own her feelings and the feelings of others.

In the group, Audrey would automatically take on the caretaker role as a means to avoid the feelings expressed by another participant. The role also helped her avoid whatever feelings this interaction had triggered in her, since she was busy trying to come up with solutions to other members' issues. She often monopolized the time by delivering detailed stories that staved off the emotions she had learned to avoid at all costs. Audrey quickly resorted to giving advice in a manner that intimated to the other members that the solutions to their problems were easy—if only they would follow her suggestions. Initially, the members did not confront these behaviors. However, over the course of the 3 years that Audrey attended the group, the pattern emerged and members reacted strongly. They would discuss their anger at Audrey in meetings that she was unable to attend. When she asked what had happened in her absence, they confronted her with their anger. She would cry, complain about the group's insensitivity (which would curtail conversation), and announce her intention to leave the group. Audrey was stymied by their anger because her actions had been the only avenue to relationships in her past. The following week, Audrey would return, apologize about her behavior and pledge to improve. Members of the group began to repeatedly confront Audrey about her inability to sit with feelings. This pattern occurred again and again.

My own reaction (strategy of disconnection) was avoidance of any confrontation that would cause this cycle, because I did not understand it and was not sure how to work with it. My own relational image of being a caretaker who focused on "needing to make things better" was triggered. I recalled a vignette about my childhood that my mother described to me when I was training at a state mental institution. In the 1950s my aunt was a psychiatrist and the director of a mental hospital in upstate New York. As the psychiatrist-in-chief, she lived in a large house on the grounds, with bars on the windows. I was 5 years old when, on a visit to see my aunt and uncle, my mother found me crying at a window. When she asked me why I was upset, I replied, "The people are so sad. I want them to feel better." Certainly, there were positive outcomes in my life that are linked to the motivation behind this relational image. However, my initial reaction in the group of avoiding confrontation was based on the mistaken idea that the anger would not make things better. I felt inadequate because I did not know how to work effectively in the group. I was afraid to confront Audrey, because I did not know if I could, in fact, make things better. I had to become aware of this triggered response and develop the different approach of encouraging the expression of anger. In this case, the expression of anger was actually a strategy of connection. When one member expresses his or her feelings of disconnection in a group, chances are that another member feels the same way and both feel connected by the revelation (Fedele, 1994).

The relational images from members' past, such as "My feelings are unimportant" or "I am insignificant," were activated so they believed that she simply did not want to listen to them. Their anger at Audrey thereby became fueled by their own past hurts. Carla did not confront Audrey openly about her inability to just sit with people's feelings. Carla's facial expressions and gestures toward me seemed to indicate that she was censoring herself due to the level of anger that she experienced. However, Carla was very vocal about her anger when Audrey was absent. When I questioned her about her inability to bring up these issues in Audrey's presence, Carla explained that Audrey would not listen and that she, Carla, could not express her anger in a reasonable way. It was too overwhelming, because its source was in her relationship with her own mother.

There was some movement in the group when a member shared that sometimes she just wanted Audrey to listen. In time, members discussed their experience of not being able to connect with Audrey around her true feelings. Audrey's behavior was aimed at avoiding difficult feelings in the group—both her own and other members'. It frightened her to face her feelings of inadequacy and vulnerability. Because Audrey did not want to engage the relational image that she most feared—"I am unlovable if I am depressed"—she had an extremely difficult time letting go of this caretaking strategy of disconnection. Paradoxically, it allowed her to avoid the disavowed parts of herself (feelings of inadequacy and loneliness) that she could not tolerate, at the same time that it contributed to her feelings of isolation and loneliness. However, when members expressed their wish to connect with Audrey around her genuine feelings and to see her as she truly was, things changed slowly. To her surprise, Audrey began to face and share those very feelings with other members in the group and found that she felt deeper connection with others and greater clarity of her own needs.

As the group leader, I was perplexed by my own dilemma. On the one hand, Audrey's extreme vulnerability was palpable, and the group's need to protect her from their anger was understandable. My own strategy of disconnection around avoiding anger colluded here. On the other hand, I recognized that people were tuning out and group process was stalling. My wish to be a good-enough therapist collided with this perception. The relational images activated for me were "I am inadequate" and "I must not hurt anyone." Whenever a member did mention Audrey's monopolization of the group or her inability to listen, Audrey often substantiated everyone's fears by crying, becoming enraged at the group, and threatening to leave. The members, having heard this tune before, would listen without comment. In the next session, Audrey would panic because no one would protest her threats to leave. I would weave my way toward an empathic comment about her ability to take people's comments home and really think about them. This response would move Audrey to discuss her dependence on the group and its importance in her life. It took time for the connection in the group to coalesce around the shared feelings of anger, isolation, and inadequacy. Slowly, the group members, recognizing both her and their own underlying strength, were able to handle all of her feelings, including anger and panic. The group would reconnect around the meaning of the group in their lives. Participants got better and better at recognizing their own patterns and avoided feelings less and less. It took repeated interactions, impasses, and working through feelings to shift Audrey's strategies of disconnection. When people could understand the strategy, they began to empathize with Audrey's need for it, without accepting or condoning it. In this empathic, though relationally challenging, setting, Audrey began to discover new strengths and capacities.

The constriction of roles based on dysfunctional relational images and their meanings from the past prompted substantial discussion in the group, particularly when the roles were rigidly maintained in current relationships. For example, avoiding feelings as a strategy of disconnection created difficulty in the group because Audrey could not simply listen and encourage other women. It impaired her ability to engage in an empathic mutual interaction. As the group members responded honestly to Audrey, they too had to overcome their own issues with anger. They challenged Audrey's views of herself and what she needed to do to remain in mutually growth-fostering relationships. This change in the equilibrium of group interaction allowed Audrey, Carla, and the other members to learn new roles and elaborate feelings that had been previously disavowed. They each began to develop a new set of relational images and to develop a fresh template for mutually satisfying relationships.

Group dynamics are always complex, and each member's relational images combine to form a multilevel matrix of interaction. Working with these images and changing each member's pattern of relationship is sometimes like trying to untangle a kite's string after flight. It has often become inadvertently knotted and intertwined because of hasty maneuvers and desperate kite-flying strategies. Each member's strategies of disconnection and relational images must be examined both within the group context and within the context of each person's experience. Audrey's strategy of avoiding feelings interlocked with the entire group's (including my own) difficulties with anger. Carla experienced an overwhelming amount of inner anger about her relationships, particularly with authority, which was evident in her tense relationships with her supervisors. Carla's attempts to keep her anger out of the group were unsuccessful. Although she made great efforts to disguise her feelings, the anger that finally emerged seemed disproportionate to the actual issue being discussed. She was aware of this discrepancy. Since Carla had chosen a profession that valued healthy interaction and a positive sense of connection, she experienced the conflict quite deeply and felt intense shame about her difficulties at work, her referral to the group, and her jarring manner in the group. She had little patience and responded with crispness.

At times, I reacted to the level of rage directed at me, as an authority figure, with intense discomfort. However, I was able to shift toward an empathic understanding with the help of Irene Stiver, Judith Jordan, and my colleagues in a weekly consultation group that I attended. Each time I presented the material from the group, I could more easily maintain this empathic stance during the next meeting. My colleagues' ability to validate and understand the dilemma between my discomfort and my wish to catalyze healthy interaction allowed me to break through strategies of disconnection and move into empathy. It is my observation that the intense feelings generated toward me, as the group leader, and the resulting feelings I experienced were often so overwhelming that a supportive consultation group was the only way to contain, tolerate, and understand them in context. I began to comprehend the profound loss that was beneath each member's anger. Each time I empathized with the reasons for her anger as a strategy of disconnection, Carla felt a bit more comfortable with her feelings. With my modeling and encouragement over time, the other members also learned to empathize with the reasons for Carla's feelings, which allowed her to move further into the experience of the anger and to examine its roots. This reassurance set the stage for members to experience anger as a *part* of the relationship rather than as an end to it. Gradually, Carla began to talk about her feelings more openly.

In the position of group leader, I appreciated that there was always a delicate balance to maintain between the expression of anger as a constructive versus a destructive force. I needed to keep a sound perspective regarding my own ability to control or manage anger in the group. I sometimes tried to diffuse the anger in the room by directing it back toward myself. Paradoxically, sometimes my attempts to control or manage anger in the group was not a movement toward safety so much as my own strategy of disconnection. I needed to remain aware of my wish to be liked or admired and to openly acknowledge my limits and blind spots to the group; indeed, I did so, many times, recognizing to group members that, realistically, there were many ways that I, as the leader, could fail. This admission had a dramatic and empowering impact on the members. On one occasion, I attempted to explain the reason for an impasse, but my words came out jumbled and barely coherent. One of the other members saw that I was having difficulty and interceded, explaining, in a very articulate way, what I had been trying to say. The whole group realized what had happened, and I acknowledged that she had said it much better than I had. Members acknowledged a whole range of feelings in response to this transaction, from disappointment to joy, and much discussion ensued. For weeks, the members good-naturedly referred to the time that I could not make sense, and we all laughed about it. This incident catalyzed members' abilities to be accepting of, and authentic about, their own feelings and insecurities. It also assisted them in negotiating both the realistic feelings of disappointment *and* the relational images regarding parental or authority figures.

CRITICAL JUNCTURE

After both Audrey and Carla had been members of the group for about a year, the pattern and tensions examined above were clear. Audrey came to group perfectly groomed in expensive clothes and talked about the concerns of her children, her thriving business, and her marriage. Issues of class were apparent, with Audrey representing a privileged upbringing and lifestyle. Her clients were people of substantial means. Her attempts to appear perfect occasionally triggered others' perception of her as entitled. Ironically, this "tyranny of appearance" was based on her insecurity and wish to be accepted, and a complex group context evolved out of it. Culturally, Audrey's Italian background contributed to her demonstrative, and, at times, overwhelming, presentation. Carla, in contrast, was severe and uncompromising in her lack of pretension. Her humble class roots had created hardship, and her current financial situation, though not precarious, was fluctuating. Although she found New England Protestants to be restrained, at the same time she was astonished by what she perceived as Audrey's torrents of emotion. All these cultural differences set the stage for tension within the group context.

Audrey's principal vulnerabilities were her insecurities in relationships and her propensity toward, and fear of, depression. Any confrontation would cause Audrey to cry, announce that she would leave, only to return to the group the following week with a great deal of anger and sadness. Each time Audrey returned to the group expressing her anger and sadness, people reacted initially with frustration, but they would move quickly to a clearer understanding of her strategies of disconnection. The empathic interaction would move her to explain her thoughts and feelings during the course of the week. She was able to empathize and agree with the other members' perceptions and announce a renewed commitment to the group. Each time this pattern emerged, Audrey's ability to hear feedback gradually improved.

Audrey would often tell stories about the downright nasty manner in which some of her very wealthy clients treated her. She attempted to avoid the deep shame her clients' treatment elicited in her. It was only when members asked why she put up with this disrespect that she could acknowledge the tremendous pain these interactions caused her. Some members became fearful of Audrey's vulnerability, tried to avoid being authentic with her, and moved into a disconnected state. Each time Audrey returned to the group the following week, she reported how she had thought about the group's input—but always with a firm, practical reason to keep these clients. She usually cited the importance of the clients and her wish to please these demanding patrons. Her feelings were left disregarded in a heap.

Carla, in a strikingly different presentation, discussed her commitment to helping others in unfortunate circumstances. She emphasized the meaning of her work and felt she did not need to focus on a financial reward. Carla's physical appearance in the group was modest; indeed, she almost disappeared into the surroundings. She continued to be deeply troubled by the paradox of her commitment to relationship and her intense anger. As described previously, Carla, after initially avoiding any expression of her anger in the group, soon became comfortable (1) expressing anger toward people outside of the group, and (2) expressing anger to group members. The validation, acceptance, and empathy she experienced in the group were critical to this transformation. Carla sincerely wanted to explore the disconnection in relationships that her anger caused and to understand the psychological experiences that had framed her images and feelings.

The tensions between Audrey and Carla culminated in one group session when it seemed as if fireworks had exploded. Audrey was discussing a particularly demeaning and abusive interaction with the husband of a wealthy client, when Carla could restrain herself no longer and suddenly become harshly critical of Audrey. With her face distorted in frustration and disgust, Carla accused Audrey of acting like a whore, prostituting and demeaning herself for money. We were all taken aback by the intensity of feeling and by the disparaging tone of this outburst. After a moment of shock, Audrey bitterly retorted that Carla had no right to judge her. She, at least, earned a decent living, whereas Carla got only pennies and annoying self-righteousness in return for her labor. She added that Carla did not even take good care of herself or of how she looked. Carla's face changed from rage to shock to pain. The muffled fury that each woman experienced in her inner world had been unleashed in this sudden outpouring. Each of them (as well as the group) was surprised by the ferocity of this interchange. At the end of the scheduled time, the group was at a standstill.

Although I floundered around and tried to say something intelligent or soothing, nothing hit the mark. Predictably, Audrey announced that she would not return to the group. She did not expect to be treated this way and was furious that I had *allowed* such a painful interchange to occur. Carla demurred, saying that she hoped Audrey would come back so that they could figure this whole thing out. Carla admitted that anger was the reason she was in the group in the first place. Their ability to articulate their positions with such clarity engaged my own relational competence. I validated and applauded Audrey's anger at being mistreated and Carla's tenacity at examining her strategies of disconnection. I also announced that I understood the reason for anger at me, as the leader, and for any sense that I might have failed them. I closed by acknowledging that it was also difficult for me to sit with these painful feelings, but that I would reflect upon the session during the course of the week, as I hoped they would. I recognized that, although anger is disturbing, it is *a part of the process of relationship* and not the end of relationship. I reminded them that I expected to see them all the following week. Finally, I thanked them in advance for hanging in there with the group and me.

Awareness of my inner reaction as the leader was critical in understanding the complex relational environment of this group. My overall concern was whether this specific interchange would have serious consequences for the long-term viability of the group. I was aware of my own paradox between connection and disconnection as a window on the group process. On the one hand, I wanted to be liked and respected as a good group therapist, and whether the group continued had a tremendous impact on that self-perception. On the other hand, the amount of rage these members expressed toward each other triggered my own avoidant strategies of disconnection. I also was aware of my sense of disconnection as a way to monitor the experience of participants. If I felt disconnected and overwhelmed, it was a strong indication that other members also felt this way. It was also important for me to remember how profoundly painful the experience of disconnection can be.

In the group, I acknowledged my discomfort, which the members experienced as validating and empathic. I also acknowledged their anger at me, as the leader, for my inability to contain the affect in the room. Both these interventions moderated the level of rage in the room without interrupting the process in the group. At the same time, my being empathic and validating the anger allowed it to remain in the group process for further work the following week. Acknowledging that, although it was difficult, I expected everyone to return and help me continue to process the feelings was a way of containing the anger within the relational context of the group. This framing of situation suggested to members that it was manageable, even as I tried to convince myself that it was. This empathic stance bypassed (1) my need to be a good therapist who was in control and could do no wrong, and (2) my wish to avoid the anger. As the leader it is my responsibility to set the stage for the possibility of mutuality in relationships. This modeling encourages empathy in members and creates the potential for a matrix of mutual empathy between and among each person in the group.

TRANSFORMATION THROUGH MUTUAL EMPATHY

A superficial look at the dynamics of the dyadic interaction indicated that both women were extremely critical of the other's lifestyle. Certainly issues of class, social status, and culture permeated this dichotomy. Yet, underlying these feelings of anger and disdain was a common bond: That is, they both felt unworthy and ineffectual in changing how certain people treated them. They were locked in self-deprecating relational images that they were not good enough. The pair of women, and the group, needed to tolerate and understand the anger within the relationship in order to get past it and comprehend the sadness, loss, and desperation underlying it. The relational–cultural model describes mutual empathy and mutual empowerment as the mutative factors in the therapeutic relationship. Mutual empathy helps catalyze the transformation of negative relational images into more empowered ones. The experience of mutuality in this relationship allowed for further transformation and growth.

Although a number of members contacted me during the week, concerned about what might happen in the group, I encouraged them to be hopeful, and everyone showed up on time at the next meeting. To Audrey's credit, she returned triumphantly to the group and, after an initial uncomfortable silence, proudly announced that she had "fired" the abusive client. To the group's amazement, she declared that Carla was indeed correct and that she, Audrey, had been prostituting herself. Audrey was empowered by Carla's empathy for her yearning and acted on the wish to be treated respectfully. This was an incredible movement on Audrey's part. In fact, members wondered for weeks whether she would find some reason or necessity to return to this client. She held firm and proudly announced each week her continued resolve. Carla, for her part, had also thought carefully about what Audrey had said. She penetrated her strategies of disconnection (anger and disdain) and recognized her own yearning for validation. Carla resolved to either get a better wage or find a different position. Movement on this front was slower for Carla than Audrey, but it was effective nonetheless.

That these two women had weathered a fierce storm with the group had created a strong bond. Together they had learned about the complexity of anger as a strategy of disconnection for each of them in her own unique way. In being empathic with each other, they could be empathic with themselves. They had created a context of mutual empathy and recognized their own yearnings. In speaking their true feelings, they could progress past them and uncover hidden parts of themselves. Audrey and Carla openly and passionately discussed their differences and similarities, and other members witnessed the interchange, totally engrossed in the process. Audrey was involved in a flashy career that focused on appearance, whereas Carla was intimidated by appearances. This was a difference, but underlying this difference was a similarity. Carla felt undervalued because she did not make much money; Audrey, because she did not feel respected. All members appreciated the paradoxes and intricacies of these dynamics, both for Carla and Audrey and for themselves. This matrix of mutual empathy became a dramatically transformative force in the group. Relational images of inadequacy formed in their past relationships changed to empowered images of tolerance and strength. At the same time, the expression of extremely intense anger became less forbidding and less dangerous to the process of relationship. They had not only survived the anger, but it had enhanced their understanding of themselves, their understanding of people in their past, their understanding of each other, and their understanding of *the process of relationship*.

Over a couple of months, Audrey and Carla began to discuss another similarity: their perception of their mothers as judgmental. They talked about the experience they both shared of their mothers "on their shoulders, watching every move" they made. They discussed how both their mothers were critical of their appearance, yet they each had developed a different strategy of disconnection. Audrey tried to achieve perfection to please her mother and to avoid the painful critical interactions. Although this strategy did not really work, it had become her trademark way of relating to herself and others. This strategy constrained her response to people-pleasing ones and diminished her capacity to be authentic. Carla, in contrast, had rebelled and had given up all hope of ever pleasing her mother. She was invested in *not* caring how her mother felt about her or how she, Carla, looked. This strategy did not work either, because Carla's longing for love and acceptance simply went underground, covered by a thick veneer of rage. Anger became a hallmark of her presentation; it constrained her interactions by infiltrating all her relationships. Both women experienced intense yearnings for the love and affection of an idealized, nurturant mother, but they each developed unique strategies of disconnection to deal with the yearnings. They also developed different relational images that were nonetheless linked by their shared experience. The empathic context of the group elicited their courage to examine and understand the complexity of their true feelings and the meanings behind their relational images. Real transformation occurred in the group for all members.

As Audrey and Carla articulated their experiences with their mothers, they each began to refine their understanding of the complexity of their relationships to their sisters. The intense anger and jealousy between these two members, we eventually learned, was rooted in their relationships to their sisters. Each sister had adapted the alternate strategy of disconnection as a protection from the mother she also experienced as critical. Carla's sister had painstakingly followed their mother's prescriptions in order to avoid feelings, just as Audrey had done. Carla had had a turbulent relationship with this "goody-two-shoes" sister. Audrey's smart sister, on the other hand, had openly rebelled against their mother's dictums about appearances. This rebellion had interfered with Audrey's sister's sense of confidence, as she had only recently, at 40, completed her doctorate in the social sciences. Predictably, until this point, Audrey and her sister had a mediocre relationship without much authentic interaction or intimacy. These realizations helped both Carla and Audrey empathize with their sisters and understand the troubled relationships they had each had with them. Both of them and the group began to consider alternate ways to handle these kinds of relationships in a manner that would enhance the potential for better connection.

The narrative of Audrey and Carla's group interaction demonstrates relational movement and mutual empowerment as experienced in this therapy group. The resolution of this critical juncture in the group process attests to the power of relationships in that process. Initially, everyone responded to the outburst of anger with discomfort and with a characteristic strategy of disconnection. Over time, as the group progressed, this authentic expression of anger, within a construct of empathic relationship, allowed for movement in the group. Anger, although unpleasant, must be considered a valuable part of relationship, rather than the demarcation of the end. Through the expression of anger, Carla and Audrey experienced authentic parts of themselves that had been constricted by relational images from their past. They were able to learn about the complexity of anger and its usefulness. This experience is also relevant to the dilemma of being real and authentic in a relationship versus responding to other people's needs. We all must find the balance between responding authentically in a given situation and, at the same time, responding in a way that is sensitive to the needs of the other person. Although the initial expression of the anger in this incident was more authentic and less empathic, the relational context of the group allowed for increments of movement toward more mutual empathic connection. Carla and Audrey each broke through their strategies of disconnection by understanding their need for them in the first place. By considering this tapestry of (1) relationship, (2) relational images, and (3) strategies of disconnection, we begin to see the complexity of the issues and feelings that these two members alone bring to a group. We can then begin to appreciate the wealth of relational material available in a group of six members. The potential for transformation of relational possibilities in a group context is truly awesome.

SUMMARY

In this vignette, Audrey and Carla reached a greater understanding of their own strategies of disconnection, their underlying relational images, and the meanings each image commands. They made substantial progress in dealing with their presenting problems and in developing better relationship skills. Both these women, as members of the group, moved through complex layers of relational images and their cognitive constructions. The particular critical juncture in the group interaction, described here, allowed all the members to achieve greater clarity about themselves, greater clarity about each other, and greater clarity about the process of relationship. The relational–cultural context of the group gave rise to this possibility of relational growth and awareness.

All the members of the group presented with relationship issues involving either personal, school, or work arenas. Since the group therapy was based on a relational–cultural model, disconnections in relationships were seen as the source of psychological problems. The goal of this group therapy was to move relationships in the group from disconnection to fuller and deeper connection. Learning these relational skills in the here-

and-now reality of the group would allow members to apply these same relational abilities to other relationships in their lives. In individual work, a fuller and deeper connection is possible only if the therapist is moved by the patient, and the patient can feel that the therapist is moved (Miller & Stiver, 1997). In group therapy, this notion expands to include all member-to-member and member-to-leader relationships. Deeper and fuller connections are possible if any member is moved by another member/leader, and they both experience that movement. There is a further deepening of relationship, since the group members/leader can also bear witness to emotional movement in the group. The possibilities for these healing interactions are increased in a group format, as are the complexities.

REFERENCES

Collins, P. H. (2000). *Black feminist thought: Knowledge, consciousness and the politics of empowerment.* New York: Routledge.

Fedele, N. M. (1994). Relationships in groups: Connection, resonance and paradox. *Work in Progress, No. 69.* Wellesley, MA: Stone Center Working Paper Series.

Fedele, N. M. (2001, February 14–19). *A Stone-centered relational approach to group psychotherapy.* Paper presented at the annual meeting of the American Group Psychotherapy Association: Diversity Matters: Exploring our Differences, Boston.

Jordan, J., Walker, & Miller, J. B. (2001, June 21). *A relational reframing of the process of change.* Paper presented at the Jean Baker Miller Summer Advanced Training Institute, Wellesley, MA.

Miller, J. B., & Stiver, I. P. (1995). Relational images and their meaning in psychotherapy. *Work in Progress, No. 74.* Wellesley, MA: Stone Center Working Paper Series.

Miller, J. B., & Stiver, I. P. (1997). *The healing connection.* Boston: Beacon Press.

Part IV

Envisioning New Models of Effectiveness and Change: Relational Practices in Institutional Settings

Although relational–cultural theory is associated primarily with clinical practice, the foundational tenets require us to examine how relationships are structured in organizations. Just as traditional models of human development have valorized separation, autonomy, and power-over methods and models as hallmarks of the healthy self, traditional models of institutional practice overrely on rigidly stratified power and unilateral control to ensure organizational effectiveness. Whether the organization is an ad hoc committee or a highly structured bureaucracy, both anecdotal and research evidence suggests that the values and mechanisms of power-over strategies and values are operative (Fletcher, Jordan, & Miller, 2000; Jaffe, 1995; Walker, 2002). The valorization of the power-over mentality is expressed in many of the taken-for-granted aphorisms about organizational functioning—from "the buck stops here," with its virtuous connotations of tough-minded responsibility, to the somewhat derisive admonitions against "letting the inmates run the asylum." At base, each of those expressions (with multiple gradations in between) signals a deeply ingrained cultural propensity to associate leadership with individual might and unilateral control. The "important people" in the organization resist influence from the less important people (Miller, 1976). Indeed, power-over is seen as the only way to achieve organizational success. It is no small surprise, then, that competitive striving often undermines organizational effectiveness. In such settings, conflict degrades into conquest, and power is used—overtly, covertly, and sometimes *unwittingly*—to ensure permanent inequality between dominant and subordinate groups.

The authors of the chapters in this section describe their involvement in projects that directly challenge this set of values and practices. These contributors work to initiate change by employing the precepts and practices of the relational–cultural model in the institutional context. In each of the cases, albeit to varying degrees, introducing relational practice was counter to the prevailing institutional culture. In addition to implementing the goals of the particular project, the authors had to counter institutional mistrust, primarily because the dominant group tended to attribute any success they had previously experienced to the effectiveness of power-over practices.

In "Prevention through Connection," Linda Hartling describes her leadership of a substance abuse task force aimed at decreasing the incidence of binge drinking in college-age women. In this chapter she challenges and reframes traditional notions about the effective treatment of alcoholism. She also demonstrates the use of nonshaming interventions for destructive drinking patterns—a model that runs counter to many traditional strategies of therapeutic confrontation in the treatment of alcohol abuse. In addition, Hartling provides a clear illustration of "waging good conflict" (Miller, 1976), demonstrating how competitive conflict can be transformed into collaborative conflict to achieve the goals of the organization.

Yvonne Jenkins describes her work with the Women-in-Prison Project, which was developed and delivered under the auspices of the Stone Center/Jean Baker Miller Training Institute. Bringing relational practice to an organization whose mission is to exercise dominative control and power over inmates presented many challenges. Jenkins describes the complex sequelae of multileveled marginalization. For example, she highlights ways in which the incarcerated women disconnected from each other, as if to reinforce the societal barriers of ethnicity, language, and culture. She also describes how the women struggle to maintain their dignity in a dehumanizing system by seeking out relationship. Jenkins focuses not only on the dynamics among the women inmates, but also on the effects of the prison system on interactions among the staff. Consistent with the principles of mutual engagement, Jenkins describes how she, too, was changed in the process of bringing change to the institution.

The young women that Elizabeth Sparks encountered in her work with incarcerated girls poignantly embody the painful realities of the relational paradox. Sparks confronts the transgenerational cycles of disconnection in young women who have experienced abuse, betrayal, and humiliation in significant relationships. Although they struggle mightily to maintain some semblance of belonging, they have learned to distrust and fear intimacy. Relational yearning, in fact, is viewed as weakness. It is in this setting that Sparks works to establish a therapeutic milieu utilizing relational–cultural principles. As the chapter unfolds, Sparks explains how she grows in her capacity to hold empathic possibilities. In this work, Sparks listens to her clients, and in so doing, not only respects them, but also encourages them toward more accountability in their relationships with others. By engaging them with respect and with the expectation of mutual influence, she demonstrates alternative models of conflict.

The authors, in each instance, are describing multileveled interventions in systems with little or no history of addressing the particular needs and concerns of women. These limited projects alone were insufficient to accomplish wholesale institutional change. But they established collaborative norms at all levels of the organization, with the institutional leadership as well as with the staff and clients groups. Equally important was the implementation—the authors embodied the practices they preached.

Unlike the proverbial revolutionaries who use domination and unilateral control to bring about "democracy," these change agents understood the necessity of being both teachers and models of relational practice. Jordan has long held that power-over is the option exercised by those who have learned to fear and distrust relationship. The authors demonstrated an alternative model of institutional effectiveness, one that is powered by empathic awareness, authentic responsiveness, and mutual respect and accountability.

It is not uncommon for scholars of relational–cultural theory to describe their hopes for changing the culture of disconnection to one that acknowledges and validates the fundamental interconnectedness of all life. This expression is not a grandiose fantasy but a lived commitment to continual learning. It is a commitment to participate in growth-fostering relationships not just in the 50-minute therapy hour, but in ways that help people experience the expansiveness of their human potential, wherever they may be.

REFERENCES

Fletcher, J. K., Jordan, J. V., & Miller, J. B. (2000). Women and the workplace. *American Journal of Psychoanalysis, 60*(3), 243–261.

Jaffe, D. T. (1995). The healthy company: Research paradigms for personal and organizational health. In S. L. Sauter & L. R. Murphy (Eds.), *Organizational risk factors for job stress.* Washington, DC: American Psychological Association.

Miller, J. B. (1976). *Toward a new psychology of women.* Boston: Beacon Press.

Walker, M. (2002). Power and effectiveness: Envisioning an alternative paradigm. *Work in Progress, No. 94.* Wellesley, MA: Stone Center Working Paper Series.

11

Prevention through Connection
A Collaborative Approach
to Women's Substance Abuse

LINDA M. HARTLING

After graduating high school as class valedictorian and a National Merit scholar, Alicia was accepted at a prestigious college, a college she believed would ultimately prepare her for a fulfilling career in medicine. With an outstanding academic record and a promising future ahead of her, no one would have predicted that this successful, self-disciplined, conscientious young woman would find herself in a hospital emergency room during her first week of college, her life on the line after a single night of heavy drinking. No one who knew her would have anticipated that she, like a growing number of college women, would land in such a state. Fortunately, Alicia was connected to a circle of caring friends who recognized the warning signs of serious intoxication. Acting quickly, these friends called 9-1-1, and Alicia was taken to the hospital where she was immediately treated for acute alcohol poisoning.

Alicia's story is one of many similar stories I have heard while working in college counseling centers. A college education remains a key component of women's efforts to overcome social, political, and economic obstacles; however, more and more women are finding their academic achievements seriously disrupted or derailed by the firsthand effects (e.g.,

197

lower academic performance, acquiring a sexually transmitted disease, physical injuries, car crashes, alcohol poisoning, etc.) or the secondhand effects (e.g., becoming a victim of verbal, physical, or sexual assault, etc.) of high-risk alcohol use and other substance abuse. A recent survey indicated that 41% of women at co-ed institutions had engaged in binge drinking (defined as four or more drinks in a row) within a 2-week period (Wechsler et al., 2002). At women's colleges, these researchers determined that the number of women engaging in binge drinking had increased 36% since 1993 and the percent of women reporting frequent binge drinking (binge drinking three or more times in the past 2 weeks) had doubled (Wechsler et al., 2002). Another study, compiling existing data available from federal sources, suggests that substance abuse, in many instances, is increasing more rapidly among women than men (Drug Strategies, 1998).

Historically the majority of individuals engaging in substance abuse has been men; consequently, most approaches to prevention and treatment have not been designed to respond to the concerns of women. However, a growing number of studies suggests that women are rapidly closing the substance abuse gender gap. More and more girls are trying alcohol, tobacco, and drugs at younger and younger ages, and more women over 60 are relying on psychoactive prescription drugs, including tranquilizers and sedatives (Drug Strategies, 1998). These trends indicate an urgent need to develop approaches to preventing substance abuse that are attuned and responsive to women's experiences and psychological development.

This chapter describes an approach to substance abuse prevention that incorporates an understanding of the issues that influence women's substance use and abuse while integrating key concepts of relational–cultural theory, as it has been developed by the scholars of the Stone Center at Wellesley College (Jordan, 1997; Jordan, Kaplan, Miller, Stiver, & Surrey, 1991; Miller & Stiver, 1997). Relational–cultural theory can be utilized as a theoretical foundation for establishing more effective methods to prevent substance abuse among women, as is seen in this example of the development of a collaborative community response to prevention. Multiple forms of connection can indeed be mobilized to reduce substance abuse among women: that is, *prevention through connection.*

SUBSTANCE ABUSE: MOVING TOWARD A RELATIONAL UNDERSTANDING

Most models of prevention are rooted in traditional theories of psychological development that define healthy development as a process of separating from relationships and becoming more independent and self-sufficient. Following these dominant theories, substance abuse is viewed individualistically, suggesting that the problem is located within the individual, who is deficient in some way—for example, ill-informed, weak-willed, immature, or easily influenced by others; or one who has poor decision-making skills, low self-esteem, no self-control, or misperceives social norms (Berkowitz, 1997; Buckman, 1995; Daugherty & O'Bryan, 1993; Perkins & Berkowitz, 1986). As a result, many approaches to preventing substance abuse emphasize teaching information or skills to increase an individual's ability to stand alone, think independently, be self-sufficient, and resist peer pressure—that is, prevention through self-sufficiency, disconnection, or separation. Individualistic understandings of substance abuse often spotlight and magnify the *dangers of relationships*. "Relational" terms have come to have negative connotations, such as "dependency," "enabling," "codependency," peer pressure," and so on. Yet recent research suggests that being in relationships—having a connection with others—can be a protective factor that reduces the risk of developing a substance abuse problem (Blum & Rinehart, 1997; CASA, 2001a, 2001b; Resnick et al., 1997). Perhaps the traditional "separate-self" models of psychological development have constricted our understanding of the complex relational dynamics that influence an individual's involvement with alcohol and other substances, thus preventing us from forming deeper understandings of these problems. Furthermore, traditional models have led us to overlook the important qualities of relationships that help reduce an individual's risk of developing a problem with drugs or alcohol.

Relational–cultural theory challenges us to bring a keen awareness of relationships into the center of our thinking about substance abuse prevention. It offers us a way to understand the complex relational disruptions and violations—for example, child abuse, sexual assault, trauma, depression, eating disorders, and so on—that can trigger or exacerbate addictions in women. Relational–cultural theory provides a template for examining alienating and isolating social–cultural conditions of sexism, racism, homophobia, and other forms of marginalization that can increase the risk of developing a substance abuse problem. In contrast, growth-fostering relationships (Miller & Stiver, 1997)—relationships characterized by mutual empathy, mutual empowerment, and mutuality—can enhance the resistance and resilience to the adversities that often precipitate the development of substance abuse-related problems or addictions (Spencer, 2000). Putting relationships at the center of our thinking about substance abuse prevention gives us a new lens through which we can review existing strategies and formulate new, more effective approaches to prevention.

WOMEN AND SUBSTANCE ABUSE: A DISEASE OF DISCONNECTION

From the perspective of relational–cultural theory, women's substance abuse can be described as a *disease of disconnection*—a disease that (1) separates and isolates a woman from essential relationships that can help reduce her risk of developing a substance abuse problem (Covington & Surrey, 1997; Finkelstein, 1996; Gleason, 1993; Markoff & Cawley, 1996; Spiegel & Friedman, 1997) and (2) separates her from relationships necessary for well-being and growth (Miller & Stiver, 1997; Spencer, 2000). This disease of disconnection is characterized by a complex interaction of factors that affect an individual's ability to overcome serious relational disruptions or adverse experiences that can trigger or intensify substance use and abuse. These factors also influence a woman's ability to find and maintain relationships that would lead her toward well-being, healing, or recovery.

Taking a relational view of women's substance abuse does not mean overlooking biological factors. Research tells us that all individuals have varying degrees of biological risk for developing a substance abuse problem and that women's physical responses to alcohol and other drugs are different from men's. For example, women become intoxicated after drinking roughly half as much alcohol as men. Women metabolize alcohol differently from men, get drunk faster, become addicted more easily, and develop health-related problems more rapidly (CASA, 1996). Relational–cultural theory leads us to pay special attention to the biological factors associated with a woman's substance abuse because these factors also affect a woman's ability to participate in the relationships that are central to psychological well-being and health (Banks, 2000).

Keeping women's unique biological risks in mind, we can begin to explore the relational–cultural dynamics associated with women's substance use and abuse. Informed by an understanding of women's psychological development and relational–cultural theory, we can explore two paths by which women become involved with drugs or alcohol: (1) to facilitate connection in response to a natural desire for connection, and/or (2) to cope with relational disruptions and violations, including traumatic experiences.

Substance Use and the Desire for Connection

Every day young women are bombarded with advertising and other media messages suggesting that personal and relational success depends on having a certain appearance or buying the right product. For decades advertisers have marketed idealized images and catchy slogans to capitalize on women's desire for connection. The alcohol industry spends an estimated $6.5 billion annually to imply, via advertising, that their products will enhance romance, intimacy, attractiveness, popularity, or sex appeal (Drug Strategies, 1998; Kilbourne, 1999). Advertisers present alcohol as a necessary accompaniment to rewarding interpersonal interactions, including romantic dates, successful social gatherings, festive celebrations, and so on. In actuality, advertisers are marketing an *illusion of connection*—the illusion that wearing the right clothes, being the right weight, drinking the right drink, taking the right pill, and so forth, can lead to satisfying, enduring relationships.

Compounding the pressures inflicted by relentless advertising, the challenge of finding connection in a culture of growing disconnection (Putnam, 2000; Walker, 1999) intensifies women's vulnerability to alcohol or drugs. Women (and likely men) learn quickly that the chemical effects of substances can diminish social inhibitions, reducing their fears of rejection and isolation in social settings. In her poignant book, *Drinking: A Love Story*, Caroline Knapp described the seductive effect of alcohol: "That may be one of liquor's most profound and universal appeals to the alcoholic: the way it generates a sense of connection to others, the way it numbs social anxiety and dilutes feelings of isolation, gives you a sense of access to the world" (1996, p. 64).

Heterosexual women are frequently introduced to the use of alcohol and drugs through their relationships with boyfriends, husbands, or fathers. Women will match the substance use behaviors of their male partners, perhaps in an attempt to strengthen bonds within these relationships (Williams, 1998). Lesbians face extremely daunting obstacles in their efforts to find connection. Confined by the real dangers of living in a heterosexist, homophobic society, lesbians have few opportunities for developing social and intimate connections beyond bars and other establishments that serve alcohol or where illicit drugs are readily available (Finnegan, 2001). In intimate relationships, the majority of women who drink says that they expect alcohol to facilitate their sexual pleasure. These women report that drinking has a positive affect on their sexuality and emotional intimacy, even though heavy drinking results in higher sexual dysfunction, a higher risk of sexual assault, and a higher risk of acquiring a sexually transmitted disease (CASA, 1994; Wilsnack & Wilsnack, 1997). In many instances, alcohol or drug use becomes entangled with efforts to find authentic relationships and fulfill the natural desire for connection.

Substance Abuse as a Source of, and Response to, Serious Disconnections

Substance abuse often contributes to many forms of serious disconnection and violations, including interpersonal conflict and interpersonal violence, family disruption or violence, physical and sexual abuse, incest, assault, and more. It is estimated that substance abuse causes or exacerbates 7 out of 10 cases of child abuse or neglect (Reid, Macchetto, & Foster, 1999). Seventy-five percent of sexual assaults reported to authorities involves alcohol consumption by the attacker, the victim, or both (Warshaw, 1988). In 70% of domestic violence cases the assailant or the victim had been drinking (CASA, 1996). In response to these harmful experiences, it is not surprising that some individuals may turn to substances to mitigate their pain and trauma. It has been shown that 90% of all alcoholic women reported being physically or sexually abused as children and that 59% of female adolescent drug users were sexually victimized (CASA, 1994). Victims of trauma or traumatic disconnections may use alcohol or other drugs (i.e., self-medication) to manage their bodies' biochemical responses to acute stress, which can persist long after a traumatic event has occurred (Banks, 2000).

In addition, substance use and abuse may provide women with a precarious but readily accessible method for coping with the profound sense of disconnection associated with depression. Stiver and Miller (1988) describe the feelings of chronic disconnection and isolation that women experience when they become depressed. Depression is the most frequent mental health disorder accompanying women's alcoholism, and women more than men develop alcoholism following depression (CASA, 1996). Women may become involved with alcohol or drugs to find relief from the ravages of depression, chronic and profound feelings of disconnection, or the effects of trauma.

Substance Abuse as a Progression of Disconnection

Women's substance abuse can be viewed as a progression of disconnection leading toward increasing isolation. Although substance use and abuse may begin as an attempt to build relationships and/or to cope with serious disconnections, these efforts can culminate in the substance becoming a woman's primary relationship—a toxic substitute for connection.

This relational perspective on women's substance use and abuse leads us to consider new possibilities for reducing and preventing women's alcohol/drug-related problems. In the remaining section of this chapter I explore a community case example, describing efforts to improve and enhance prevention programming at a women's college.

CREATING A CONNECTED COMMUNITY: A CASE OF PREVENTION THROUGH CONNECTION

As Alicia's story illustrated at the beginning of this chapter, there are increasing concerns about women's substance abuse on college campuses.

In response to these concerns, I was hired at a woman's college to develop an alcohol/drug education program for students, faculty, and staff. The administration of the college was supportive of efforts to develop programming based on an understanding of women's psychological development, as proposed by relational–cultural theory. After conducting a campus-wide assessment, in collaboration with key members of the community (i.e., students, staff, administration, and faculty), I began the process of implementing a program based on the principles and practices of relational–cultural theory. This approach was designed to facilitate greater community connection and reduce disconnection and isolation, two factors that can increase women's risks of developing a substance abuse problem. Three key components were included: (1) making interpersonal connections, (2) strengthening community connections, and (3) building interscholastic connections.

Making Interpersonal Connections

The first priority at this academic institution was to provide a more effective and consistent response to individual students engaged in high-risk substance abuse-related behaviors (e.g., binge drinking, acute intoxication, illegal or abusive drug use, etc.). Rather than directing these students to large group educational experiences, which are commonly used on many campuses, this program began to provide students with free, private, confidential alcohol/drug consultations. In these consultations I offered students specific, personally relevant information for assessing their level of risk, and I helped them identify a range of choices that would reduce their risk of experiencing an alcohol/drug-related problem (Daugherty & O'Bryan, 1993). Although this information often appeared to be helpful, my key goal in these consultations was to establish an interpersonal connection with an individual who recently experienced an alcohol or drug-related problem. The following stories are examples of the consultations I conducted over a 2-year period with students exhibiting high-risk drug or alcohol behaviors.

"Yasmine's" Story

Yasmine, a first-year, first-semester international student, was referred to me for consultation after she had been taken to the campus infirmary by other students who became concerned about her intoxication and vomiting following a party. When we met several days after this event, Yasmine appeared to be extremely ashamed, and she expressed deep regret for her behavior. She said that she had never drunk alcohol before coming to this country, because it was prohibited by her Islamic religious beliefs. However, in an effort to meet and "fit in" with American students (a natural desire for connection), she had joined some acquaintances at a small, impromptu "party" on campus, where drinking was the center of the social activity. Reflecting the behaviors of other students at the party, Yasmine quickly consumed "three" shots of vodka. Although she thought she had made a "moderate" drinking choice, compared to students who were consuming large quantities of alcohol, after a while she became extremely sick and could not stop vomiting. Her friends eventually decided to take her the infirmary.

Sending Yasmine to a large-group alcohol program following her experience would have overwhelmed her with shame and left her feeling publicly disgraced or humiliated (Hartling, Walker, Rosen, & Jordan, 2000; Jordan, 1989). Fortunately, the privacy of a one-on-one consultation appeared to mitigate her intense feelings of shame and facilitated an open conversation about her experience. It allowed her to disclose and examine personal factors that contributed to her severe reaction to drinking, including being exhausted that day, missing dinner prior to the party, feeling highly stressed, and being of a physically petite stature. In addition, Yasmine began to reveal some of the challenges of being an international student and a Muslim.

"I just wanted to be like other students in this country. I wanted to be with them and show that I could do what they do to have fun, which meant drinking," Yasmine declared, "but now I am mortified by what's happened. My family would be so angry and ashamed of me."

"I understand that you feel ashamed of what has happened, especially because it would disappoint your family," I said to her. "At the same time, it seems to me that wanting to meet and get along with others is an important goal when you are in a new community and a new country. In fact, I think it is a smart thing to do. The challenge is to find ways to join with others without losing yourself, without sacrificing what is important to you."

After empathizing with and affirming her desire to create relationships in a new environment, we began to explore some of the challenges of connecting across cultural differences at this particular college. Yasmine acknowledged the dangers of attempting to build relationships with others by matching their high-risk behaviors, such as drinking or drug use. She also recognized that the pressures she felt to assimilate into the U.S. college culture had led her to neglect developing connections with other international students who have similar religious beliefs and values. In addition, it appeared that her efforts to conform to mythical U.S. standards of independence and self-sufficiency had led her to distance herself from her primary support system: her family. These were some of the relational conditions and dilemmas precipitating Yasmine's high-risk drinking experience. Naming these dilemmas was the first step in her recovery from this experience. By the end of our consultation, Yasmine had decided that she would get involved with some of the international student groups on campus and meet with the advisor for Muslim students to begin the process of finding a community of individuals who would support and share her values and religious beliefs. In addition, she identified ways she might connect with U.S. and other non-Muslim students without compromising her religious practices or personal values.

"Julie's" Story

Julie was a first-year student who referred herself for an alcohol/drug consultation. She was anxious and upset as a result of an experience she said had occurred during the prior weekend. She explained that she had been drinking at a party hosted by a fraternity at a neighboring academic institution. At the party, she drank too much and decided to lie down on a couch in a quiet area of the fraternity. Although her memories of what happened after that were foggy and confused, she tearfully described becoming aware that sometime during the night, one of the fraternity members had had intercourse with her. In distress, she exclaimed, "I never meant to hook up with anyone at the party! I only had a few drinks. I never intended to get drunk and let someone take advantage of me!" Clearly she held herself completely responsible for drinking too much. However, I noted that she had no way of estimating the amount of alcohol in the drinks mixed at the fraternity, and she had no way of knowing if the mixed drinks contained other drugs that could have incapacitated her.

As Julie described her state of distress and the fraternity event, I realized that she was trying to cope with a traumatic experience, quite possibly a sexual assault, which would require services beyond a single consultation. Yet Julie's only motivation for scheduling an appointment was to acquire information about how she could prevent this type of experience from ever happening again, to regain a sense of safety and control. In addition to honoring her desire for information about alcohol, I wanted to create a compassionate connection with Julie that would encourage her to consider additional services for treating her trauma or possible sexual assault, which could trigger future involvement with drugs or alcohol.

To address Julie's concerns, I began our consultation with an examination of factors that influence response to alcohol and risk of developing an alcohol-related problem. This process allowed Julie to understand some of the complex biological factors that might have contributed to her unintended level of intoxication, for example, being tired, not eating, consuming mixed drinks with an unknown amount of alcohol content, consuming drinks containing other drugs, and so on (Daugherty & O'Bryan,

1993). This discussion of specific, concrete, personally relevant information appeared to have a calming effect on Julie. Her self-contempt eased as she began to consider the many factors that may have contributed to her becoming incapacitated, including the possibility that other drugs were mixed into her drink. She also began to realize that no matter how drunk she was, no one had a right to violate her sexually. By the end of the consultation, Julie agreed to arrange a meeting with a staff member in the counseling center to address her experience of trauma. Through consultation empowered by connection, Julie was able to take action and seek the services she needed to fully understand and recover from her alcohol-related traumatic experience.

"Felicia's" Story

Felicia was a sophomore who referred herself for an alcohol/drug consultation after hearing about the start of this free, confidential service on campus. Meeting Felicia in a waiting area, I was surprised to find that she had brought her boyfriend, "Terry," to the meeting. Terry was a senior from a neighboring academic institution. He and Felicia had been dating for a number of months. During the meeting, Felicia said she did not drink alcohol or use drugs, but that she had a growing concern about Terry's drinking. Although Terry did not drink regularly, every time he drank he would get extremely drunk. Felicia was worried about what might happen to him whenever he became highly intoxicated. She was particularly concerned because her feelings for Terry were growing stronger. Without any hesitation, Terry responded, "I think Felicia is right. I don't drink very often, but when I drink, I can't stop and I know this scares Felicia. I know she thinks I'm going to have an accident or get seriously injured in some way when I'm out drinking with my friends. I also know my drinking is affecting our relationship." He said that Felicia was very important to him, and he recognized that his pattern of drinking to get drunk was problematic, even though it had not yet resulted in any other obvious problems (e.g., academic difficulties, disruptive or aggressive behavior, property damage, etc.).

Much of the literature on substance abuse describes the dangers of "enabling" substance abuse behaviors within relationships. Felicia's actions reflected the positive side of enabling someone she cared about to seek information before he experienced a major difficulty. Because of my understanding of relational–cultural theory, rather than presaging the risks of codependency in a relationship where one person is drinking, I was able to honor the strength of Felicia and Terry's relationship that made it possible for them to seek help early. Supported by their love for, and connection to, each other, both Felicia and Terry were able to explore their individual risks of developing an alcohol-related problem. In particular, Terry was able to examine his family history of alcohol problems and higher-than-average tolerance for drinking large quantities of alcohol. Without defensiveness or denial, Terry acknowledged the signs of increased risk that could lead to a serious alcohol problem if he continued his current pattern of drinking. Finally, the consultation concluded with a discussion of low-risk choices that would reduce Terry's and Felicia's risks of ever experiencing an alcohol-related problem during their lives (Daugherty & O'Bryan, 1993).

Several weeks after this consultation, I made a follow-up phone call to Felicia to ask about how things were going. "Terry's quit drinking and decided to focus his energy on his academic work and career goals," she said, "This has taken the strain out of our relationship and we enjoy being with each other more than ever."

"Stephanie's" Story

Stephanie was referred after having been taken from campus to a local hospital for observation as a result of acute alcohol poisoning. When I met with Stephanie, she was initially angry about being required to attend an alcohol/drug consultation; nevertheless, she gradually warmed up and began to describe some of the events that had led up to her acute intoxication. Stephanie was a senior studying economics, one semester away from graduating, but she was currently having academic difficulties that were threatening to derail her graduation. She stated that she did not drink alcohol regularly and had never had any other experiences of acute intoxication, but this was not the first time she had tried to get extremely drunk. She also said she did not have a family history of alcohol problems, a history of trauma, or eating disorders. However, as she began to feel more comfortable with me, she explained that for the past 3 years she had absolutely "hated" her college experience. Unlike other students at this particular college who had many financial advantages that allowed them to attend an expensive private academic institution, Stephanie revealed that she was from a struggling, working-class family and had had to negotiate enormous financial obstacles to attend college. Despite the success of being accepted at a prestigious academic institution, she described how the class difference between her and the majority of her peers had led her to experience a profound sense of disconnection, alienation, and, ultimately, isolation. Consistent with her lifelong efforts to "pull herself up by the bootstraps" and be completely self-supporting and self-sufficient, she explained that she had never talked to anyone about her desperate unhappiness and feelings of isolation. Binge drinking appeared to be one method she used to cope with her feelings when they became intolerable.

"A group of students from my dorm went on a trip to Acapulco together over spring break, staying in a fancy hotel, sitting on the beach, drinking and dancing all night long," said Stephanie, in disgust, "As usual, I had to work during spring break. Even if I wanted to, I couldn't afford to go with them. I just stayed here and got drunk."

If I had focused only on Stephanie's binge drinking, I would have missed the most significant factor contributing to her drinking: class shame (hooks, 2000). Fortunately, relational–cultural theory promotes attunement to issues of class, race, gender, and sexual orientation that can become sources of intense pain and alienation. Tuning into Stephanie's concerns allowed me to validate the reality of her struggles and work with her to develop a plan of action that would help her move on to finish her degree with out relying on binge drinking. First, Stephanie agreed to schedule an appointment with a therapist in the counseling center to discuss her feelings about her college experience. Then she identified a trusted college staff member with whom she could share her concerns. Finally, by the end of the consultation, she suggested that she might eventually share her experience with a college administrator to help the college administration understand the unique challenges that a student from a working-class family encounters while working and living in a college community where most of students have upper-class privileges.

Strengthening Community Connections

The second priority for implementing prevention through connection at this academic institution was to mobilize and strengthen community relationships as a part of the effort to address alcohol/drug problems. One specific example of strengthening community connections was the formation of a collaborative committee of campus representatives to examine substance abuse issues. Appointed and supported by the college administration, I was placed in charge of organizing and chairing a collaborative Alcohol/Drug Advisory Committee.

To form the committee, I recruited individuals representing a diverse sampling of campus constituencies: a member of student government, a student who was a resident assistant in the dorms, the associate director of health services, the campus health educator, a campus police officer, a faculty member, a representative of counseling services, and a head-of-house from the residential system. After the committee was established, the college administration asked it to revise the existing alcohol/drug policies to maximize student safety, while upholding state and federal laws and avoiding unnecessary, intrusive measures. Additionally, the administration assigned the committee the task of developing "understandable *and* enforceable policies" that would hold students accountable while moving them toward constructive changes in behavior.

As the chair of this committee, with a background in relational–cultural theory and practice, I viewed its formation as a critical opportunity to create a connected community response to substance abuse. Having participated in past committees that had devolved into endless, emotionally charged, adversarial discussions of alcohol policies, I was committed to using relational practices to facilitate constructive discussion of these issues. These relational practices included (1) "listening others into voice," which involved actively encouraging committee members to openly share their views; (2) promoting mutual empathy by developing a bidirectional sense of understanding among committee members; (3) encouraging mutual empowerment by promoting the sense that each and all members of the committee have an impact on the committee's thinking and work together; and (4) waging good conflict—approaching conflict in a way that leads to positive change (Miller, 1976, 2002).

From the beginning, the members of the committee voiced diverse and sometimes contentious concerns. Student representatives expressed fear that revising the policies would automatically result in students losing individual privacy and rights. Campus faculty and staff representatives expressed concerns about student safety and the college's legal liability. Campus police and residents staff were particularly concerned with the enforceability and consistency of the proposed revised policies. Fortunately, understanding relational–cultural theory allowed me to view conflict as a necessary and beneficial part of fostering the growth of the participants' connection, rather than acting as an impediment (Miller, 1976).

As difficult as it was, as a group we encouraged a "bring-it-on early" approach to dealing with conflict, actively encouraging members to respectfully voice their concerns and objections to proposed revisions of the existing alcohol/drug polices. This, combined with other relational practices, allowed the group to move through arduous disagreements. For example, after a year of work, on the day before the committee planned to deliver its revised alcohol/drug policy to the college administration, a student representative, "Lisa," shocked the other members of the committee by declaring, "We can't give this to the administration. Students will not accept the new policy. They will rebel! It will be a disaster! I won't let this happen!"

"Wow, Lisa, I can tell you are really concerned," I commented, focusing on Lisa. "I'm very glad that you have brought this to our attention now before we take the policy to the administration." Rather than discounting, challenging, or denying her 11th-hour objection, members of the committee joined me in expressing empathy for Lisa, and with this shared perspective we began to explore her concerns.

"During our year together, we have worked through a number of problems with our proposed alcohol/drug policy," I said. Did we miss something that has come to your attention?"

Downshifting her heightened emotions, Lisa identified one aspect of the policy that the rest of the committee acknowledged might be confusing to some members of the campus community. Lisa pointed out that rushing to finalize the policy too quickly could trigger an unnecessary negative reaction from students, which would completely distract them from seeing the positive aspects of a policy that was actually an improvement. Acknowledging Lisa's concerns, the committee formulated a new process for implementing their revised alcohol/drug policy that would allow them to make adjustments to the policy, if necessary, during the upcoming year. Specifically, they decided that the revised policy would be used as an interim policy during the first year of its implementation, which would be considered a transition year. During this transition year, students, faculty, and staff would have the opportunity to give the committee additional feedback about the effectiveness and clarity of the revised policy. After a 1-year trial period in which policy could be adjusted, the final version of the policy would be implemented in the second year. Lisa agreed that this extended process of implementing the policy would be a useful way to respond to her concern and still move forward.

Lisa's 11th-hour concern could have derailed the committee's efforts. Instead, the committee's collective relational practice led to a more resilient response to a member's sincere concern. Ultimately, acknowledging and validating Lisa's objection enabled the committee to improve the process for implementing the policy. Instead of breaking apart in the face of a last-minute conflict, committee members were able to draw upon their relational skills to address Lisa's concern and create an effective solution. Responding to, rather than reacting to, Lisa's concerns facilitated her reconnection with the group's collaborative work.

Building Interscholastic Connections

A third component of my efforts to implement a program of prevention through connection involved building relationships with professionals working with substance abuse at other academic institutions. After a series of tragic alcohol-poisoning deaths on campuses around the country, many college professionals were motivated to join together in their efforts to prevent these and other alcohol/drug-related problems. With the support of the administration, I represented the college at meetings with representatives from various institutions of higher education to discuss campus alcohol and drug issues.

One example of making an interscholastic connection to prevent and reduce alcohol/drug problems on campus involved joining other professionals from neighboring college campuses to formulate a shared agreement to improve practices in response to high-risk drinking (Task Force on Underage and Problem Drinking, October 1998). Over the course of many months, this group of representatives developed a list of shared goals that formed a cooperative agreement on methods of reducing and preventing high-risk drinking behaviors on all campuses in the surrounding metropolitan area. Although a few of these goals could not be applied at a women's college (e.g., managing behaviors at fraternities), many of the goals could be readily utilized, including:

- Promoting and increasing availability of alcohol-free programming on campus.
- Reducing alcohol advertising on or near campus.
- Ensuring the training and support of residential staff.
- Encouraging the development of peer support services and programs.
- Offering faculty training to help members learn how to identify problem behavior and provide appropriate intervention.
- Establishing methods to communicate and cooperate regularly with local police and municipal authorities.
- Increasing partnerships with area campuses, public officials, police services, surrounding neighborhoods, the business community, students, alumni, parents, and secondary schools.
- Continuing the planning and evaluation of prevention efforts.

In addition to creating a collaborative agreement, building relationships and working in connection with professionals from other academic institutions allowed all of us to benefit from the collective wisdom developed through sharing and discussing our individual and community efforts to prevent the growing problem of substance abuse.

Assessing the Impact of Prevention through Connection

As most people in the field of prevention know, it is difficult to completely or accurately assess the degree to which a program has been effective or ineffective. However, there were indications that the prevention-through-connection efforts described in this chapter were exerting positive effects:

1. None of the students referred for an alcohol/drug consultation due to acute intoxication repeated their behavior.
2. Compared to prior semesters, incidents of acute intoxication were cut almost in half.
3. Students who attended alcohol/drug consultations encouraged

other students to utilize the confidential services, and voluntary consultations thereby increased.

4. Members of the advisory committee continued to meet to discuss concerns and finalize revisions of alcohol/drug policies, which were then successfully implemented.

5. The development of an interscholastic cooperative agreement provided a national model of colleges working together to address alcohol/drug-related problems.

PREVENTION THROUGH CONNECTION IS FOR EVERYONE

This chapter describes some of the new possibilities and opportunities that became evident when we applied a relational–cultural approach to preventing high-risk alcohol/drug-related behaviors on a women's college campus. It highlights the components of a connected community response— *the practice of prevention through connection*—to address high-risk alcohol and drug use: creating interpersonal connections, strengthening community connections, and building interscholastic connections. Fortunately, more and more people are recognizing that connections and collaborations are essential for effective, comprehensive prevention efforts. A recent article in the *American Psychologist* (Weissberg, Kumpfer, & Seligman, 2003) stresses that "children will benefit most when families, schools, community organizations, health care and human-service systems, and policymakers work together to strengthen each other's efforts rather than working independently to implement programs" (p. 427).

Still, one of the greatest advantages of prevention through connection has yet to be stated. Whereas many approaches to prevention *must* be implemented, orchestrated, and coordinated by specially trained professionals, *everyone can actively participate in prevention through connection every single day!* Relational–cultural theory suggests that whenever we promote, provide, or develop growth-fostering relationships, we are, in effect, reducing the risk that individuals will develop a problem with alcohol or drugs—so *anyone* can participate in this process. Rather than falling solely under the province of the "experts," the practice of prevention through connection is an inclusive approach. Parents, family members, teachers, professors, peers, administrators, community service providers, supervisors, employers, and others who build growth-fostering relationships are simultaneously practicing behaviors that can reduce the risk that an individual will seek out and/or choose to engage in high-risk alcohol and drug behavior. Furthermore, people who build growth-fostering relationships provide a key ingredient of resilience, which allows individuals to overcome hardships, trauma, and adversities that can trigger substance abuse problems (Hartling, 2003). Ultimately, we may discover that connection is the most powerful component of effective prevention.

REFERENCES

Banks, A. (2000). PTSD: Brain chemistry and relationships. *Project Report, No. 8.* Wellesley, MA: Stone Center Working Paper Series.

Berkowitz, A. D. (1997). From reactive to proactive prevention: Promoting an ecology of health on campus. In P. C. Rivers & E. R. Shore (Eds.), *A handbook of substance abuse for college and university personnel* (pp. 119–139). Westport, CT: Greenwood Press.

Blum, R. W., & Rinehart, P. M. (1997). *Reducing the risk: Connections make a difference in the lives of youth* [Report]. Minneapolis: Division of Pediatrics and Adolescent Health, University of Minnesota.

Buckman, R. B. (1995). *The other side of the coin. Drug prevention programming in higher education* (5th ed.) [FIPSE manual]. Washington, DC: U.S. Department of Education.

CASA. (1994). *Rethinking rites of passage: Substance abuse on America's campuses* [Special report]. New York: Columbia University Press.

CASA. (1996). *Substance abuse and the American woman* [Executive Summary]. New York: Columbia University.

CASA. (2001a). *National Survey of American Attitudes on Substance Abuse VI: Teens* [Special report]. New York: Columbia University.

CASA/ (2001b). Shoveling up: The impact of substance abuse on state budges [Special report]. New York: Columbia University.

Covington, S. S., & Surrey, J. L. (1997). The relational model of women's psychological development: Implications for substance abuse. In R. W. Wilsnack & S. C. Wilsnack (Eds.), *Gender and alcohol: Individual and social perspectives* (pp. 335–351). New Brunswick, NJ: Rutgers Center of Alcohol Studies.

Daugherty, R., & O'Bryan, T. (1993). *On campus . . . talking about alcohol and drugs* [Training manual]. Lexington, KY: Prevention Research Institute.

Drug Strategies. (1998). *Keeping score 1998: Women and drugs: Looking at the Federal Drug Control Budget* Washington, DC: Author.

Finkelstein, N. (1996). Using the relational model as a context for treating pregnant and parenting chemically dependent women. *Journal of Chemical Dependency Treatment, 6*(1/2), 23–44.

Finnegan, D. (2001). Clinical issues with lesbians. In *A provider's introduction to substance abuse treatment for lesbian, gay, bisexual, and transgender individuals* (pp. 73–77). Rockville, MD: U.S. Department of Health and Human Services.

Gleason, N. (1993). Women and prevention: Lessons from an alcohol education program. *Work in Progress, No. 3.* Wellesley, MA: Stone Center Working Paper Series.

Hartling, L. M. (2003). Strengthening resilience in a risky world: It's all about relationships. *Work in Progress, No. 103.* Wellesley, MA: Stone Center Working Paper Series.

Hartling, L. M., Walker, M., Rosen, W., & Jordan, J.V. (2000). Shame and humiliation: From isolation to relational transformation. *Work in Progress, No. 88.* Wellesley, MA: Stone Center Working Paper Series.

hooks, b. (2000). *Where we stand: Class matters.* New York: Routledge.

Jordan, J. V. (1989). Relational development: Therapeutic implications of empathy and shame. *Work in Progress, No. 39.* Wellesley, MA: Stone Center Working Paper Series.

Jordan, J. V. (Ed.). (1997). *Women's growth in diversity: More writings from the Stone Center.* New York: Guilford Press.

Jordan, J. V. (1999). Toward connection and competence. *Work in Progress, No. 83.* Wellesley, MA: Stone Center Working Paper Series.

Jordan, J. V., Kaplan, A. G., Miller, J. B., Stiver, I. P., & Surrey, J. L. (1991). *Women's growth in connection: Writings from the Stone Center.* New York: Guilford Press.

Kilbourne, J. (1999). *Can't buy my love.* New York: Simon & Schuster.

Knapp, C. (1996). *Drinking: A love story.* New York: Dial Press.

Markoff, L. S., & Cawley, P. A. (1996). Retaining your clients and your sanity: Using a relational model of multi-systems case management. *Journal of Chemical Dependency Treatment, 6*(1/2), 45–65.

Miller, J. B. (1976). *Toward a new psychology of women.* Boston: Beacon Press.

Miller, J. B. (1988). Connections, disconnections, and violations. *Work in Progress, No. 33.* Wellesley, MA: Stone Center Working Paper Series.

Miller, J. B. (2002). How change happens: Controlling images, mutuality, and power. *Work in Progress, No. 96.* Wellesley, MA: Stone Center Working Paper Series.

Miller, J. B., & Stiver, I. P. (1997). *The healing connection: How women form relationships in therapy and in life.* Boston: Beacon Press.

Perkins, H. W., & Berkowitz, A. D. (1986). Perceiving the community norms of alcohol use among students: Some research implications for alcohol education programs. *International Journal of the Additions, 21*(9/10), 961–976.

Putnam, R. (2000). *Bowling alone: The collapse and revival of American community.* New York: Simon & Schuster.

Reid, J., Macchetto, P., & Foster, S. (1999). *No safe haven: Children of substance-abusing parents* [Special report]. New York: Center on Addictions and Substance Abuse at Columbia University.

Resnick, M. D., Bearman, P. S., Blum, R. W., Bauman, K. E., Harris, K. M., Jones, J., Tabor, J., Beuhring, T., Sieving, R. E., Shew, M., Ireland, M., Bearinger, L. H., & Udry, J. R. (1997). Protecting adolescents from harm. *Journal of the American Medical Association, 278*(10), 823–832.

Spencer, R. (2000). A comparison of relational psychologies. *Project Report, No. 5.* Wellesley, MA: Stone Center Working Paper Series.

Spiegel, B. R., & Friedman, D. D. (1997). High-achieving women: Issues in addiction and recovery. In S. L. A. Straussner & E. Zelin (Eds.), *Gender and addictions: Men and women in treatment* (pp. 155–165). Northvale, NJ: Aronson.

Stiver, I. P., & Miller, J.B. (1988). From depression to sadness in women's psychotherapy. *Work in Progress, No. 36.* Wellesley, MA: Stone Center Working Paper Series.

Task Force on Underage and Problem Drinking. (1998, October). *Cooperative agreement: Boston area colleges and universities*. Boston: Boston Coalition.

Walker, M. (1999). Race, self, and society: Relational challenges in a culture of disconnection. *Work in Progress, No. 85*. Wellesley, MA: Stone Center Working Paper Series.

Warshaw, R. (1988). *"I never called it rape": The* Ms. *report on recognizing, fighting, and surviving date and acquaintance rape*. New York: Harper Row.

Wechsler, H. (1996, July/August). Alcohol and the American college campus: A report from the Harvard School of Public Health. *Change*, pp. 20–25, 60.

Wechsler, H., Lee, J. E., Kuo, M., Seibring, M., Nelson, T. F., & Lee, H. (2002). Trends in college binge drinking during a period of increased prevention efforts. *Journal of American College Health, 50*(5), 203–217.

Weissberg, R. P., Kumpfer, K. L., & Seligman, M. E. P. (2003). Prevention that works for children and youth. *American Psychologist, 58*(6/7), 425–432.

Williams, K. (1998). *Learning limits: College women, drugs, and relationships*. Westport, CT: Bergin and Garvey.

Wilsnack, R. W., & Wilsnack, S. C. (Eds.). (1997). *Gender and alcohol: Individual and social perspectives*. New Brunswick, NJ: Rutgers Center of Alcohol Studies.

12

Toward Relational Empowerment of Women in Prison

YVONNE M. JENKINS

The previous chapters have powerfully illustrated the clinical benefits of relational–cultural theory within the 50-minute individual therapy
hour. This chapter illustrates the theory's versatility by shifting to its value
as a tool toward the relational empowerment of an institution and, ultimately, to society-at-large. Toward this end, I focus on the application of
relational–cultural theory in the Women-in-Prison Project of Wellesley
College (Duff, García-Coll, Miller, & Potter, 1995), an endeavor designed
in the early 1990s to reduce the incidence of recidivism among women at
a minimum security prerelease prison in the Northeast. It was also hoped
that this project would expand our understanding of the life experiences
of women in prison, in addition to introducing growth-fostering relationships to these women.

THE WOMEN-IN-PRISON PROJECT

The Women-in-Prison Project was supported by the Massachusetts Committee on Criminal Justice and the Stone Center for Research on Women
at Wellesley College. The project was developed to address the relational,
cultural, and developmental needs of incarcerated women at a minimum
security prerelease prison, and to document themes in their psychosocial

experiences with the intent of improving existing services and reducing recidivism. Of particular interest was the identification of ways in which women can develop empowering relationships that encourage connection in prison. Special attention was paid to (1) how women from different racial and ethnic groups experienced incarceration from a relational perspective, and (2) the ways in which diversity issues and personal history impacted relational development, so that more effective programs focused on prevention and rehabilitation could be developed. Last but not least, attention was given to incarcerated women's relationships with their children.

RELATIONAL-CULTURAL THEORY

Relational–cultural theory, also known as the Stone Center theoretical approach, is the basis for relational–cultural therapy, a clinical approach that focuses on defining and understanding connections and disconnections that either foster or restrict relational development. Relational–cultural theory acknowledges the centrality of relationships in women's lives. It also contends that the psychological well-being, growth, and development of women are outcomes of mutually empathic relationships (Jordan et al., 1991; Miller, 1976). Thus, optimal growth and development are thought to occur through movement *toward* relationship. Rather than viewing self-sufficiency and personal gratification as the primary motivators in people, this model, according to Jordan and Dooley (2001), acknowledges the primacy of our need to establish connections with others; it "suggests a shift away from what has been primarily a psychology of the individual, or separate self, to a psychology of connection or relatedness" (p. 2). The relationale for this approach is to move from disconnection to connection through the medium of relationship. The Women-in-Prison Project took this concept into a rigid institutional context to promote positive connection between incarcerated women and prison personnel at the following levels: (1) policymakers and administrators, (2) staff (i.e., supervisors, security, line staff, etc.), and (3) community care and aftercare staff. This goal of connection was promoted via four project segments:

1. *Three conferences* were sponsored by the Stone Center for Developmental Services and Studies and the Massachusetts Committee for Criminal Justice in 1994, in an effort to integrate relational–cultural approaches into the care, treatment, and aftercare of women in prison. These conferences introduced participants to the relational–cultural theory of women's psychological development and emphasized the importance of this perspective when ad-

dressing the needs of women in prison. The first two conferences provided an unprecedented opportunity for a diverse cross-section of senior administrators, policymakers, and prison employees (e.g., security, supervisors, line staff, trainers, mental health providers) from the Massachusetts Department of Corrections to discuss the needs of incarcerated women from a relational–cultural perspective. The third provided a similar opportunity for community care and aftercare personnel.

2. *Needs assessments* were conducted via focus groups and interviews with the women and staff.

3. *A training program* based on relational–cultural theory was developed as a more effective form of intervention with this population.

4. *The training model was then piloted and evaluated* by the Department of Corrections administration, staff, and the incarcerated women themselves.

I participated in developing, piloting, and evaluating the training model elaborated later in this chapter.

BEHAVIORAL PROFILE AND RELATIONAL NEEDS OF WOMEN IN PRISON

Prison systems have typically been designed with the needs of incarcerated men in mind. However, the behavioral profile and relational needs of incarcerated women differ from those of incarcerated men (Fine et al., 2001; Women-in-Prison Project, 1995). Fine and colleagues (2001) and Duff and colleagues (1995) assert that women are the fastest growing segment of the prison population, with a rate that doubles that of men. Women more often serve time for nonviolent offenses in which they are accessories to crime, whereas men are often convicted of violent crimes. In addition, women more often report a higher incidence of physical and sexual abuse and suicidal thoughts. African American women and Latinas account for a significant percentage of the current population of incarcerated women. As such, the current demographics have broad implications for understanding the multiple relational needs of women in prison, particularly women of color. For example, Potter (1994) found that cliques develop along racial or cultural lines; (1) the ability to speak Spanish is a prominent source of connection for Puerto Rican women, and (2) African American women expected African American staff to advocate on their behalf. When asked to choose an important relationship inside the prison, another outside prison, and to describe both in terms of mutuality, a higher percentage of African Americans knew their current friend in prison before the current incarceration, compared to Latinas or whites; this finding suggests a higher degree of perceived mutuality in relationships developed prior to the current incarceration. Another important relational need was suggested by visitation patterns. All white women and 92% of Latinas reported receiving regular visitors, whereas only 67% of African Americans reported regular visitors. Potter summarized:

> Male friends were the most frequent visitors (63%), followed by female friends (45%), and then relatives for all ethnic groups. However, [Latinas] reported different members of the extended family more often, including brothers, sister-in-laws, and brother-in-laws, compared to White and African American women. (p. 10)

The Women-in-Prison Project (Duff et al., 1995) observed that despite the struggles of incarcerated women, many maintain a meaningful relational context in their lives. Women were observed to be more verbal more often with prison staff than their male counterparts, and they exhibited a wider range of emotion. In addition, needs assessment interviews with women more often found them to be primary caregivers of families, including the elderly and children of minority age. The majority (75%) was composed of mothers with an average of two children, and some still had primary custody. Of those who had given up their children to the state (14%) or for legal adoption (2%), a priority for most was regaining custody. This priority was also true for some of the women whose children were in the care of fathers (24%) or other relatives (34%). Sadly, most children had not only been separated from their mothers but appeared to be separated from siblings as well, since mothers reported that their children were not living together. Mothers found it extremely important to maintain relationships with their children, were very concerned about the children's overall well-being, and about what they, as incarcerated mothers, were modeling for their children. Finally, most women with adult children found them to be a major source of emotional support.

Incarcerated women also reported more health concerns than men. This higher incidence may have been associated with the centrality of relationships in women's lives. For instance, expressed needs for health education about AIDS, CPR, and first aid may have been indicative of desires to take appropriate precaution in sexual relationships, and to take more effective care of self and others.

In respect to vocation and education, women prisoners tended to have lower job-related and academic skills than their male counterparts. In fact, Fine and colleagues (2001) assert that a disproportionate number of the incarcerated are undereducated. It is understandable, then, that most participants in the project expressed aspirations to advance their educational and vocational skills. These needs seem to have important relational implications as well. For instance, the Women-in-Prison Project reported that prior to incarceration, some women had had no opportunity to invest in their own development. The time spent in prison was also the *first* time some women had lived alone, and the *only* time they were not responsible for taking care of others. Unfortunately, this finding suggests that prison might have been *a refuge* for some women. These reports may also be associated with frequent reports of abuse among incarcerated women, and the fact that women are often accessories to crime, perhaps in an effort to take care of, or to win the approval of, another. From a relational perspective, this finding is disturbing in that it suggests the absence of positive connection to the self and others. Restoring and building such connection was central to the purpose of the Women in Prison Project.

THE TRAINING MODEL

In an effort to meet a variety of work-related needs of the staff along with the relational and multicultural needs of the incarcerated women, a training model was developed by the Women-in-Prison Project for all levels of the Department of Corrections staff. This model applied relational–cultural theory, including my concept of *embracing diversity* (Jenkins, 1993), to daily staff-to-staff and staff-to-inmate interactions. The overarching goals of training were to:

1. Increase safety for staff, incarcerated women, and the public.
2. Reduce stress by facilitating a better understanding of women's psychological development.

As part of the efforts to reach these goals, participants were informed about the relational–cultural theory, what the process of embracing diversity fundamentally involves, and cultural factors that lend contexts to the life experiences of many incarcerated women.

Incarcerated Women's Group

The population of incarcerated women in the facility consisted of African Americans, white, Latina, and others (i.e., French/Indian, Portuguese, Cape Verdean). Three of the women chose not to identify their racial or ethnic group. Several women participated in the incarcerated women's group: three whites and four Latinas. It is unclear why there were no African American participants or participants from the other racial and ethnic groups.

Line Staff Group

The line staff group included a total of 11 participants: ten women and one man. Three of the women were contract service workers. Two were African American, six were white, and three were Latina. There was an average of one or two participants at each session, with the low attendance attributed to competing, work-related priorities (e.g., the need for adequate coverage, a required week-long training seminar, emergencies, etc.). Eight of the participants completed the training program.

Supervisors' Group

Initially, there were eight white participants in the supervisors' group, two women and six men. Ongoing participation was a particular challenge for this group. Without explanation, the two women arrived halfway through the first session, completed it, and never returned. One male participant dropped out of training after completing half of the sessions. Trainers were subsequently informed that he had been granted an extended leave of absence; no further details were offered. A change in the work schedule of another participant prevented his completion of training. Therefore, only three participants completed the training, and two completed half the training. In addition, preparation for a national site certification review conflicted with the training dates. This upcoming evaluation caused supervisors, in particular, to feel conflict over the time allotted for training.

FORMAT

Participation in training was voluntary, although line staff and supervisors were encouraged to do so by the superintendent of the Department of Correction. The format of training included 2-hour sessions spaced over 6 consecutive weeks. Three groups were trained, two composed of staff and one of incarcerated women. Supervisors met in one group, whereas line staff—those responsible for monitoring the daily activities of prisoners—met in the other. All three groups received similar training, which consisted of didactic material, experiential opportunities, and vignettes. However, appropriate modifications were made to fit the needs of each group.

The sessions with staff were more comprehensive than those with incarcerated women, with whom the training focused on facilitating a practical knowledge base about relational–cultural theory and promoting the development of growth-enhancing relationships among the group members as well as with other incarcerated women. Sessions with incarcerated women emphasized self-understanding and transformation via their relationships in prison and with others in the outside world.

Participants in both groups were invited to observe their own behavior between sessions in relation to the topic areas of training. Staff were also asked to observe the behavior of the incarcerated group members. Participants in both groups were encouraged to share their observations first in dyads and then with the entire group to stimulate role playing and discussion. In each session, didactic material was presented in short segments that were informed by participants' daily experiences. Each session included vignettes based on actual occurrences at prison. At the close of each session, a handout was distributed with instructions on what to observe, and participants were asked to record their observations on 3" × 5" cards. They were also encouraged to share their observations at subsequent training sessions to stimulate problem solving via discussion and roleplaying.

CONTENT

A description of each training segment follows.

Session 1: Health Relationships and Women's Development

This session focused on the women's psychological development, the centrality of relationships in women's lives, and characteristics of healthy relationships.

Session 2: Connection, Disconnection, and Violation

Connection, disconnection, and violation were defined. Participants reflected on their understanding of how these concepts related to their own experiences. Staff participants also began to achieve an empathic understanding of the roles of connection, disconnection, and violation in the lives of many of the women in prison. In addition, characteristics of dysfunctional families and strategies for disconnection were identified.

Session 3: Disconnection and Violation

Because of the prevalence of relational violation and abuse in the lives of incarcerated women, causes of posttraumatic stress disorder (PTSD) and its behavioral manifestations were presented, as was a relational perspective of alcoholism and substance abuse. Finally, effective ways to interact with women suffering from these disorders were presented, including indicators of dangerous behavior and appropriate deescalation techniques.

Session 4: Valuing Diversity

In this session, the value of diversity was explored by increasing participants' awareness of relational images, attitudes, and behaviors that embrace diversity and how major social realities (e.g., racism, sexism, classism) devalue diversity. This session also sought to increase awareness of the diversity within the prison population and how this diversity informs the expression of connection and disconnection. Although valuing diversity was presented as a separate topic, it was appropriately integrated into all of the training segments.

Session 5: Conflict Resolution

Inmate conflict and the relational reframing of anger were the foci of this session. An open and positive attitude toward conflict and related skill building were fostered, and the presence of conflict as an opportunity for resolution and healthy relatedness was emphasized.

Session 6a: Relationships in the Workplace

Version "a" of session 6 was conducted for staff and supervisors and focused on professionalism and team building in an effort to increase connection and support among line staff, supervisors, and administrators.

Session 6b: Relationships among Women in Prison

Version "b" of session 6 focused on helping incarcerated women to improve their relationships with one another, staff, and significant others. Relevant vignettes focused on gaining more awareness of relational patterns and effective problem solving were used.

PRESENTING CONCERNS OF INCARCERATED WOMEN

The presenting concerns of the incarcerated women participants included the desire of Puerto Rican group leaders and participants to communicate with one another in their first language, Spanish, the language of their emotions; in turn, the white women felt threatened by this request, expressing anxiety and suspicion that negative comments would be made about them without their knowledge and would lead to their exclusion or disconnection from the group. After discussing this issue for a while, the decision was made to translate the training concepts into Spanish.

This decision proved to be a critical juncture in training; all participants engaged in a more meaningful manner. English-speaking participants became more eager to learn Spanish and were able to laugh at themselves in the process of doing so. Furthermore, mutuality was achieved via the process of embracing a linguistic difference, a key source of diversity. Accordingly, participants said they developed a deeper trust of one another, empathy with those who are different, and deeper appreciation for diversity.

Another concern that surfaced for this group was the desire for further education. There was a broad variation in the educational levels of the participants, and their needs ranged from those of the preliterate level to completion of the GED or college programs. Some women also expressed the desire to receive job and employment training while in prison, to learn how to reintegrate themselves into society.

Several women expressed the desire to increase their personal awareness through counseling and psychotherapy. Some women even stated how counseling had helped them deal with various problems. Those with substance abuse issues who had engaged in counseling had found it especially helpful.

A final concern that surfaced for this group related to issues of power. Frustration was expressed over participating in a program that sought to build self-esteem, only to return to their living units where they would likely be "brought down" by line staff. The women did not perceive the line staff to be informed about the program's goals, and they wanted to feel more respected by the correctional officers. This included a desire to have their addictions viewed as illness instead of criminal behavior. These concerns highlighted a realistic and complex dilemma related to power differentials among incarcerated women, the staff who are responsible for their supervision and public safety, and the professionals who are entrusted with their care or training.

The relational–cultural theory offers an important alternative to the oppressive power-over stance of traditional theories, in that it applies a power-with approach to intervention that is intended to increase the connection that is so conducive to growth-fostering relationships (Jenkins, 2000). This approach fosters "a power that grows, as it is used to empower others" (Miller & Stiver, 1997, p. 16) while respecting those boundaries that permit effective rehabilitation (e.g., institutional rules and regulations; basic dignity of each incarcerated woman as an individual).

CRITICAL JUNCTURES OF THE TRAINING

Line Staff Group

Initially, line staff workers were concerned about expressing their thoughts and feelings freely in the work environment without a threat of retribution. Some were also concerned about improving the quality of their relationships with coworkers and incarcerated women. A critical juncture of the training, initially, was to proceed with training despite the low number of participants for each session, thereby communicated the unconditional importance of the intervention while honoring the availability of those who chose to attend.

Supervisors' Group

The supervisors were initially skeptical about the content of the training, what it might reveal about their attitudes toward various aspects of human diversity, and whether or not such knowledge would be of any practical value to their interactions with coworkers and incarcerated women. A critical juncture of the training was the choice to include an exercise to sensitize participants to what it feels like to be in the minority in contrast to the majority.

As previously mentioned, except for the first session, all participants in the supervisors' group were white males. It was stunning to observe their recognition of how differently being in a minority versus the majority made them feel. As part of the majority, they felt more secure and powerful, whereas in the minority position, they felt powerless, helpless, alone, and alienated. This difference inspired them to reflect on their relationships with incarcerated women with more empathy and to identify areas for improvement. It was also moving to hear supervisors report how they used awareness gained from this exercise outside of the workplace, with family, friends, and others. In addition, they became aware of sources of diversity between themselves and other whites that pertained to gender and marital status. Attention was also given to the attitudes and beliefs concerning race and other sources of difference to which supervisors had been exposed in childhood and adolescence.

MAJOR RELATIONAL THEMES

Despite their diversity, most of the incarcerated women who participated in this project shared developmental experiences filled with violation, isolation, and disconnection. Some had left their families of origin prematurely in response to early parentification, other abusive treatment, significant loss, and emotional inaccessibility of parents. García-Coll and colleagues (1998) suggested that these factors might have placed these women at "high risk for substance abuse which can lead to criminal behavior, problems with the law and ultimately incarceration" (pp. 16–17). The cycle of disconnection continued well into adulthood in that several women had also been exposed to violence as adults. Most were serving time for crimes (i.e., prostitution, drug possession, theft) committed in conjunction with dysfunctional relationships. The women had commonly perceived these relationships as means of winning love or approval.

Other relational themes surfaced during conversations with these women. Relationships were critical mechanisms for coping with loss and separation from loved ones, especially children. Maintaining connection to family, extended family, and friends was extremely important to them. In addition, most of the women wanted to improve their relationships with other incarcerated women, to experience mutual empathy in their relationships with staff, and to leave the prison with more autonomy than when they entered it. The goal to increase self-awareness, expressed by many women, suggested a desire to nurture a more positive and intimate relationship to the self than was experienced prior to their incarceration.

Relational Images

Relational images portray the pattern of our relational experience—our explanations of *why* we are the way we are. The images embody what each of us expects to happen in future relationships as they unfold (Miller & Stiver, 1998, p. 40). Such images become the framework by which we determine who we are, what we can do, and how worthwhile we are (p. 75). If we feel heard and understood; if we hear and understand others; are motivated to act, and feel more worthwhile and more connected, then our relationships are experienced as empowering encounters. An absence of these conditions leads to disconnection, self-condemnation, and a pervasive sense of powerlessness.

Relational images that surfaced for incarcerated white women initially included the assumption that Spanish-speaking women and other marginalized cultural groups were sources of threat. These perceptions were initially shared by some staff persons. Some of the women also associated *being loved and approved of* with *the necessity to engage in risky and illegal behavior*.

Both prisoners and some of the line staff, supervisors, and administrators perceived that their peers could not be trusted with intimate aspects of their relational experience. The critical power-over stance that line staff initially assumed with incarcerated women often seemed to be influenced by relational images of the women as inferior, needy, and more trying than male prisoners. Incarcerated women were also perceived as "criminals" who need to be punished rather than as persons who are ill (e.g., addicts, alcoholics) or disenfranchised and in need of rehabilitation and support. The relational images held by staff concerning conflict were discouraging, in that these perceptions were associated with impasses and great difficulty. Conflict was believed likely to worsen if simply named or acknowledged.

Relational images of psychologists were primarily positive. Most agreed that psychologists are needed, helpful, and make the difference between life and death in some people's lives.

In another vein, the staff's relational images of the prison as a workplace had a profoundly negative tone. It was seen as a place that "sucks one dry," often leads to mental health leaves, lacks cohesion, and is generally unsupportive.

Strategies of Disconnection

Emotional disengagement, role playing, and the replication of old interactions and family dynamics that prevent one from participating in the present are familiar strategies of disconnection (Miller & Stiver, 1997). Although these strategies are protective attempts to prevent further wounding or violation, they also prevent real connection to others and are thereby tactics *for staying out* of relationships. Emotional disengagement was used by some staff to cope with what they perceived as the overwhelming neediness of incarcerated women: "I know they [line staff] treat inmates like shit. . . . It's so tough to work with them [the inmates]. Sometimes you just want to get down on their level to fight it out, but you know that's not meeting their needs" (Potter et al., 1994, p. 2). The staff's display of emotional disengagement and role playing were perceived by incarcerated women as disrespect that was "demeaning and demoralizing" and capable of destroying whatever self-esteem a woman had worked hard to achieve while in prison (García-Coll et al., 1998).

The emotional complexity of role playing as a means of job security is evident in the following statement by a staff person: "I hate this job. . . . [The] big dilemma for me is keeping my mouth shut. I see so many things that aren't being done, or are being done and are useless . . . I have to keep my mouth shut to keep my job security" (Potter, 1994, p. 9).

Replication was also evident and linked to staff hopelessness about opportunities to enhance their effectiveness: "there is no time to do [team building] . . . [it] can't be pulled off. . . . Shift by shift [you] take care of yourself, and hopefully the next shift does the same."

External Factors That Influence Relational Development of Women in Prison

A variety of high-risk factors appeared to be external to the relational development of the incarcerated women who participated in the project, even though no standardized assessment of relational development was used. These included family stress, trauma, and related substance abuse. For example, Duff and colleagues (1995) reported that 37% of the sample had not lived with their parents as children; 79% reported having been sexually and/or physically abused as children, and 55% had left home at the age of 16 or younger. There were no differences between African Americans, Latinas, and white women in the reported incidence of these factors. Seventy percent of project participants reported involvement in an abusive relationship as adults; 79% were abused as children; more than a third of the participants reported a history of substance abuse (i.e., 41% to drugs and 30% to alcohol, p. 8).

Twenty-seven of the women in the sample were white, 12 were African American, and 12 were Latinas. No definitive conclusions about socioeconomic backgrounds of the women were offered by García-Coll and colleagues (1998). However, almost half of the white and African American women were high school graduates, whereas less than half of the Latinas were of the same status. Furthermore, a higher percentage of the Latinas was born outside of the United States. Low achievement, as reflected in education attainment, work histories, and job skills, appeared to be an outcome of participants' experiences in the absence of appropriate interventions. Moreover, the power-over stance assumed by the dominant culture in the United States in relation to the treatment of African Americans, Latin Americans, and those from economically poor backgrounds, and the differential responses to this dynamic (influenced by ethnocultural values and other sources of diversity), contribute to the varying patterns of connection, disconnection, and violation associated with relational development.

Duff and colleagues (1995) asserted that for incarcerated women, maintaining relationships, especially with children, is a means of coping with separation and loss. They also suggested that policies that support punishment, versus those that support rehabilitation, make a difference in the relational experiences of incarcerated women. Punishment deters connection, whereas rehabilitation might promote connection.

Observed relational differences between groups of incarcerated women may also serve as practical indicators of need for the programs that serve this population. For example, white women often reported substance abuse that predated incarceration. This finding suggested a need for more substance abuse prevention and treatment programs for this population. African American women had fewer visitors and postrelease housing resources than other women in the sample, suggesting a need for addressing the breakdown in vital primary support systems prior to their release. Linguistic challenges experienced by Latinas and inadequate understanding of their culture on the part of supervisors and line staff suggested a need for ESL (English as a second language) programs, bilingual supervisors and staff, as well as other linguistically and culturally appropriate services.

Critical Developments That Facilitated or Impinged on the Intervention

Even though some group dialogue in Spanish between Latinas and white women was an outcome of the white women's insecurities, a critical development that facilitated that important shift was the leaders' responsiveness to the white women's interest in learning to communicate with the Latinas in Spanish. This combination of interest and responsiveness seemed to increase trust between the two groups and to influence the Latinas to feel more valued by the resulting increase in connection. Another critical development in the intervention occurred between supervisors during Session 4 (on embracing diversity). Members of the all-white male group made poignant connections between their own life and work experiences of being in the numerical minority (e.g., the only white male present; the only nonathlete present) and those of women of color and the poor.

Sessions 1 (on healthy relationships and the relational development of women) and 4 were critical interventions for the line staff. Participants expressed appreciation of the leaders who valued their ideas and permitted them to define their own experiences. They reported that the training had heightened their morale by improving their relationships with one another and increasing their hopefulness about the future.

How My Participation in This Project Affected Me

My experience as a staff member of the Women-in-Prison Project and a trainer was moving on several levels. Indeed, it was an honor and a privilege to work with two of the founding scholars, Jean Baker Miller and Janet L. Surrey, along with several other brilliant women psychologists, educators, and community activists committed to shaping and realizing the principles of relational–cultural theory. The Women-in-Prison Project was a cutting-edge endeavor that brought a very progressive alternative to the field of corrections. As such, it provided me with one of my first opportunities to collaborate thoughtfully in defining the cultural dimension of this theory via preparing a conference presentation for prison administrators and staff, collaborating on the training manual, and working as a trainer.

Working on this project has proved to be one of several unforgettable experiences of my life that has transformed my initial subjective stance of anger and futility about social problems to a more objective, active, hopeful, and productive stance regarding social change. In addition, I was stretched to practice mutuality, to see those we trained as well as myself in a more authentic manner.

Even though I was not directly involved in leading focus groups with the women, my collaboration on the project increased my empathy with them and expanded my understanding of how relational and cultural factors had impacted their development and continued to affect their plight as prisoners. My collaboration on the project also enhanced my awareness of how low staff morale, as a systemic problem, promotes disconnection in the prison setting as well as ways to confront and change this key area. Finally, my participation in this project offered valuable insight into how intervention based on relational–cultural theory has the capacity to promote the rehabilitation, rather than the punishment, of women in prison.

CONCLUSION

Of course, a substantial power differential exists between incarcerated women and the prison staff. Since the restriction of personal liberty is fundamental to society's concept of punishment and rehabilitation and deemed necessary and acceptable, is it practical or even possible, then, for mutual empowerment to be nurtured in prison settings?

From the relational–cultural perspective, mutual empowerment is both possible and necessary to achieve with women in prison. The power-with approach to relationships increases relational connection "in which each person can feel an increased sense of well-being through being in touch with others and finding ways to act on thoughts and feelings (Surrey, 1991, pp. 46–47). As Miller and Stiver (1997) have emphasized so insightfully, *mutual empowerment unlinks the concept of power from the concept of domination*. Mutual empowerment is achieved via honoring the strengths of women as well as their strategies of disconnection. "Through mutually empowering interactions, people can find the 'power to do,' to act effectively in the world" (Miller & Stiver, 1997, p. 47). Professionals *and* incarcerated women *do* benefit from mutually empowering relationships. Traditional paradigms for working with incarcerated women increase separation and disconnection. The relational–cultural paradigm offers an important shift toward increased connection that values and enlarges each person despite status or other significant sources of diversity.

The capacity of the relational–cultural approach to facilitate the transformation of troubled individual and family relationships has been known to therapists and other mental health practitioners for more than two decades. Since the inception of the theory in the early 1980s, application of this approach has broadened considerably to include organizations, institutions, and multisystems (Fletcher, 1999; Meyerson & Fletcher, 2000; Walker, 1999; Walker & Miller, 2001). The Women-in-Prison Project applied the Stone Center approach to a minimum security prison setting by hosting conferences, focus groups, and training. This project served as a progressive and innovative development in the life of an ailing institutional system—it was a breath of fresh air that facilitated connection through an atmosphere of inclusion, a sense of renewal, and possibility. Even though funding limitations did not allow the project to be renewed, those who collaborated so tirelessly on it continue to hope and trust that their work positively touches the lives of those who participated in the intervention.

REFERENCES

Duff, K. M., García-Coll, C., Miller, J. B., & Potter, M. (1995). *Meeting the needs of women in prison: Diversity and relationships*. Wellesley, MA: Stone Center for Developmental Studies and Services.

Fine, M., Torre, M. E., Boudin, K., Bowen, I., Clark, J., Hylton, D., Martinez, M., "Missy," Roberts, R., Smart, P., & Upegui, D. (2001). *Changing minds. The impact of college in a maximum security prison*. New York: The Leslie Glass Foundation.

Fletcher, J. (1996). Relational theory in the workplace. *Work in Progress, No. 77*. Wellesley, MA: Stone Center Working Paper Series.

Fletcher, J. (1999). *Disappearing acts: Gender, power, and relational practice at work*. Cambridge, MA: MIT Press.

Fletcher, J. K., Jordan, J. V., & Miller, J. B. (2000). Women and the workplace: Applications of the psychodynamic theory. *American Journal of Psychoanalysis, 60*(3), 243–261.

García-Coll, C., Miller, J. B., Fields, J. P., & Mathews, B. (1998). The experiences of women in prison: Implications for services and prevention. In *Breaking the rules: Women in prison and feminist therapy* (pp. 11–27). New York: Haworth Press.

García-Coll, C., Surrey, J. L., Buccio-Notaro, P., & Molla, B. (1998). Incarcerated mothers: Crimes and punishments. In C. García-Coll, J. L. Surrey, & K. Weingarten (Eds.), *Mothering against the odds: Diverse voices of contemporary mothers* (pp. 255–274). New York: Guilford Press.

Jenkins, Y. M. (1993). Diversity and social esteem. In J. L. Chin, V. De La Cancela, & Y. M. Jenkins, *Diversity in psychotherapy* (pp. 45–64). Westport, CT: Praeger.

Jenkins, Y. M. (2000). The Stone Center theoretical approach revisited: Applications for African American women. In L. C. Jackson & B. Greene (Eds.), *Psychotherapy with African American women: Innovations in psychodynamic perspectives and practice* (pp. 62–81). New York: Guilford Press.

Jordan, J. V., & Dooley, C. (2001). *Relational practice in action: A group manual.* Wellesley, MA: Jean Baker Miller Institute Project Report No. 6.

Jordan, J. V., Kaplan, A. G., Miller, J. B., Stiver, I. P., & Surrey, J. L. (1991). *Women's growth in connection: Writings from the Stone Center.* New York: Guilford Press.

Meyerson, D. E., & Fletcher, J. K. (2000). A modest manifesto on shattering the glass ceiling. *Harvard Business Review, 78*(1), 126–127.

Miller, J. B., & Stiver, I. P. (1997). *The healing connection: How women form relationships in therapy and in life.* Boston: Beacon Press.

Potter, M. (1994). *Discussion of staff interviews at MCI-Lancaster.* Unpublished manuscript, Women-in-Prison-Project, Wellesley College.

Sommers, E. K. (1995). *Voices from within: Women in conflict with the law.* Toronto: University of Toronto.

Surrey, J. (1991). "What do you mean by mutuality in therapy?" In J. B. Miller, J. V. Jordan, A. G. Kaplan, I. P. Stiver, & J. L. Surrey (Eds.), Some misconceptions and reconceptions of a relational approach. *Work in Progress, No. 49.* Wellesley, MA: Stone Center Working Paper Series.

Walker, M. (1999). Race, self, and society. *Work in Progress, No. 85.* Wellesley, MA: Stone Center Working Paper Series.

Walker, M. (2001). When racism gets personal: Toward relational healing. *Working Paper, No. 93.* Wellesley, MA: Stone Center Working Paper Series.

Walker, M., & Miller, J. B. (2001). Racial images and relational possibilities. *Talking Paper, No. 2.* Wellesley, MA: Stone Center Talking Papers Series.

13

Relational Experiences of Delinquent Girls
A Case Study

ELIZABETH SPARKS

Adolescence is a period of significant growth and development. For girls, it is a time that necessitates reconciliation between their sense of self and the societal definition of what it means to be a woman. Jean Baker Miller, in her seminal paper entitled "The Development of Women's Sense of Self," describes the conflict that adolescent girls experience during this period in their lives:

> [A girl's] sense of self as an active agent—in the context of acting within a relationship and for the relationship—has been altered to some degree all along by a sense of a self who must defer to others' needs or desires. However, at adolescence she experiences a much more intense pressure to do so. Her sense of self as developed so far now faces a more serious conflict with the external forces she confronts. The question is how she will deal with this conflict. (Jordan, Kaplan, Miller, Stiver, & Surrey, 1991, pp. 20–21)

Relational–cultural theory posits that adolescent girls tend to alter their internal sense of self in their efforts to deal with this conflict. They seek to become a "being-in-relation," which means developing identities where all of the self becomes integrated in complex ways and in increasingly complex relationships (Miller, Jordan, Kaplan, Stiver, & Surrey, 1991).

Relationships in which girls bring all of themselves into the connection can be positive and growth enhancing. Relationships become growth-fostering when there is mutual empathy and mutual empowerment. There is a feeling of "zest" within the connection, as well as a sense of empowerment to act within the relationship. Each individual gains knowledge about self and other, and develops a sense of worth when their thoughts and feelings are recognized and acknowledged. As a result, each feels a greater sense of connection within the relationship, and a desire for more connection with others (Miller & Stiver, 1997).

The case study presented in this chapter focuses on the complex interactions that occur in the relational lives of delinquent girls and presents a therapeutic group intervention designed to increase relational skills. The eight-session psychoeducational group intervention, based on relational–cultural theory, provided the girls with information about relationships, relational skills, and coping resources. The primary goal of this intervention was to facilitate an examination of the girls' relationship strategies.

In this chapter, I present information from the psychological literature on the relational lives of delinquent girls. To provide a broader context for the group intervention, I then discuss the external factors that influenced the treatment process. Next I explore the relational themes that emerged during the group sessions and highlight critical junctures that illustrate the movement that occurred as the girls worked through these themes. The chapter concludes with recommendations for conducting relational practice within the context of a correctional facility for delinquent girls.

THE RELATIONAL LIVES OF DELINQUENT GIRLS

Most girls who have been adjudicated delinquent by the courts have experienced relational disappointments and disconnections throughout their lives. Those who become involved in the criminal justice system are most frequently brought to court for status offenses (Chesney-Lind, 1987, 1997). These offenses include a wide range of behaviors that constitutes violations of parental authority, such as truancy, running away from home, being in need of supervision, and behaving incorrigibly. It is not unusual for girls involved in the juvenile justice system to have difficulty getting their emotional needs met. Their relational lives are often characterized by interpersonal conflict with family members, teachers, correctional staff, and peers. Many of these girls come from homes where chronic disconnection and relational violations are normative. Studies suggest that running away from home is largely spurred by extremely difficult family situations (e.g., where sexual, physical, and/or emotional abuse has occurred). These girls also report receiving limited support from the close friends, teachers, or relatives who are in a position to aid them (Fejes-Mendoza, Miller, & Eppler, 1995).

By the time young girls become incarcerated, they have experienced numerous disruptions in their lives. Typically, they have undergone removal from family, friends, and home communities, sometimes for years, often with only minimal contact with significant people in their lives. They live in situations where consistency in relationships is difficult to maintain because they, and the other residents in correctional facilities, are transitory. The girls also experience conflictive relationships with staff in the facilities where they are incarcerated or detained, making it difficult for them to form solid attachments with the only caretakers they may have for the next 2 or 3 years. Yet, despite these difficulties, most of these young women remain in search of close, nurturing relationships and approval from others (Bowers & Kline, 1983; Ginsberg, 1981).

The literature suggests that delinquent girls have three areas of need: (1) the need for respect, (2) the need for improved family relationships, and (3) the need to learn more effective ways of resisting the sexist, racist, and generally negative effects of the culture, while learning positive ways of staying true to themselves in their relationships (Belknap, Dunn, & Holsinger, 1997). Girls who become involved in delinquent behaviors seem to be struggling with a myriad of relational issues that cause them distress and pain. They are searching for someone to believe in them, and they long for respect from parents, friends, teachers, police officers, social workers and institutional staff (Pipher, 1994). The girls also want to improve relationships with family members, particularly with their mothers. Yet, most are ambivalent, feeling both intense love for their mothers along with intense feelings of anger and disappointment. Their ways of responding to these feelings are generally ineffective and contribute to their becoming involved in antisocial, delinquent behavior.

Robinson and Ward (1991) term these ways of coping with life stress "survival strategies." They state:

> From the perspective of the African American adolescent woman feeling overwhelming despair and hopelessness, employing a "quick fix" [defined as such behaviors as pregnancy; drug use and trafficking; dropping out of school; running away] to cope with life's exigencies may seem both necessary and pragmatic. (p. 95)

Through the lens of relational–cultural theory, we can understand these strategies as efforts to remain connected to others in the face of repeated relational disconnections. The central relational paradox occurs when a person's yearnings for connection are met with sustained and chronic rejections, humiliations, and other violations (Miller, 1988). The girls feel an intense yearning for connection at the same time that they perceive relationships as dangerous. In order to connect in the only relationships available, they must find ways to keep more and more of themselves hidden. They struggle to protect themselves against further woundings and rejections by not representing themselves authentically. Indeed, girls will often alter themselves to fit with what they believe are the wishes and expectations of others. However, these alterations, in effect, only serve to distance them from others (Miller, 1988).

Most delinquent girls have developed relational images that characterize relationships as being unsafe. These girls attempt to create safety by connecting only with a small number of carefully selected peers. Once they have identified the other person as a friend, however, they often are willing to participate in behaviors that they really do not want to enact in an effort to stay in connection. At times, they may even tolerate mistreatment to forestall losing the relationship. Thus, relationships pose a challenge for delinquent girls and are an important area for treatment intervention.

THE APPLICATION OF RELATIONAL–CULTURAL THEORY

Relational–cultural theory helps us better understand many of the issues inherent in the complex relational lives of delinquent girls. According to the theory, relationships that are not mutual or empathic lead to disconnection, which can have an adverse effect on girls' psychological development. Being in a mutual relationship means feeling heard, seen, understood, and known (Jordan, 1986). It means that both parties are equally invested in developing a level of intimacy and trust within the relationship that each would allow to be seen and known fully. Given delinquent girls' relational experiences and their histories of victimization, we can assume that they have been involved in few, if any, mutual relationships.

According to relational–cultural theory, the overall effect of being in long-term relationships that do not promote mutual empowerment is the construction of restricted and distorted images of relational possibilities. These constructed images further limit the individual's ability to act within connection, to know his or her own experience and to build a sense of worthiness. Jean Baker Miller (1988) has noted that chronic disconnections occur when an individual is unable to represent his or her experience fully in relationship and when the other person is unresponsive to his or her needs or pain. Furthermore, disconnection becomes problematic when the other person in the relationship does not allow him or her to participate in shaping the ongoing interaction.

Relational–cultural theory posits that when we feel the threat of isolation as both children and adults, we will try to make connection with those closest to us in any way that appears possible. We try to construct some kind of an image of self and other that would allow entry into relationships with the available people. In essence, we twist ourselves into a person who is acceptable in nonaccepting relationships. To do this, we must move away from, and redefine, a large part of our experience—particularly those parts that we believe will not be acceptable to the other person.

Miller (1988) states that whenever the only people available for connection have threatened, or actually carried out, disconnections and violations of a young woman's experience, such as when abuse has occurred, she will be unable to represent the truth of her experience both within her immediate relational context and on the larger scene. Anger is often the byproduct of this sort of violation of self experience, and of long-term threats to connection. Thus, when a young woman has experienced a lifetime of actual or threatened disconnections, she is fearful of abandonment and feels angry and ambivalent about making connections with others.

In providing clinical services to delinquent girls, we would expect to find not only histories of problematic interpersonal relationships with significant others, but also efforts to maintain relationships in the face of repeated actual or threatened disconnections. We can also anticipate that these girls have developed strategies to maintain relationships that make it necessary for them to hide or distort key aspects of who they are. Clearly, this situation is problematic for their development and psychological well-being and requires clinical interventions to address it.

DESCRIPTION OF THE INTERVENTION

Relational–cultural theory served as the theoretical foundation for the development of a psychoeducational group intervention, entitled "Understanding Relationships with Ourselves and Others," for incarcerated delinquent girls. The group had the following objectives: to help participants (1) gain a more comprehensive understanding of the nature of their interpersonal relationships, both within the residential facility and with family and friends; (2) recognize and better understand the structural forces in society that impact the lives of girls and women in adverse ways; and (3) critically evaluate the strategies they use to cope with problematic situations in their lives.

The girls who participated in the intervention were incarcerated at a residential facility in a suburban community. They ranged in age from 13 to 17 years old. For some of the girls in the group, this was their first residential placement; for others, however, it was their third or fourth placement within a 2- to 3-year period. Approximately 39% of the girls placed at the facility had a history of offenses against another individual; however, no sex offenders or offenders with histories of extreme violence were committed to this facility. Eighty percent of the girls came from urban environments. In general, about 48% of the girls who are placed in the facility at any given time is white, 28% is African American, 22% Hispanic, 2% Asian, and the rest are from "other" ethnic minority groups. Fifty percent of the population comes from two-parent households, and less than 44% has gone beyond the ninth grade in public school. A full 50% of the girls in this facility has a history of academic and learning problems.

The group met weekly for eight sessions that included structured activities and discussions in four general areas: (1) the larger societal context, (2) relational and communication skills, (3) the influence of the past on current behaviors, and (4) coping strategies and their effect on relationships. The exercises were drawn from books by Carrell (1993), Khalsa (1996), and Berman (1994). (See Table 13.1 for an outline of the sessions.) A total of eight girls was referred for the group intervention; however, at any given session, there were usually only five girls in attendance (due to medical appointments or unexpected discharges).

EXTERNAL FACTORS THAT IMPINGED ON THE THERAPEUTIC RELATIONSHIP

It is important to present the institutional context surrounding the intervention. The girls' incarceration was the principal external factor that affected the treatment process in the group. They were involuntary clients, in the sense that they were required to attend the group as a condition of their incarceration. The girls earned points for cooperating with the therapeutic components of the program, and doing so was perceived positively by their caseworkers and the legal authorities. The girls generally tried hard to cooperate so that they could remain in good standing both within the facility and the juvenile justice system. At times, however, they resented their incarceration and the treatment interventions in which they were required to participate. They would become angry and despondent during group sessions and have difficulty focusing on the material being discussed.

It is always challenging to treat involuntary clients; it generally requires a great deal of patience, empathy, and relational skill on the part of the clinician. It was essential to acknowledge and respect the girls' feelings about their incarceration, but doing so needed to be balanced with a fo-

TABLE 13.1. Outline of Sessions

Session number/title	Activities
1 The Social World of Girls	Positive Relationships Video: *Beyond Killing Us Softly: The Strength to Resist*
2 Who Am I?: Self-Esteem and Identity	Highest Hopes/Deepest Fears (Carrell) Fish for a Thought (Carrell) Knowing Yourself (Khalsa)
3 Self-Awareness	What I Value (Khalsa) What Are My Values? (Khalsa) Self-Esteem Inventory (Khalsa) T-Shirt Exercise (Carrell)
4 Getting in Touch with Feelings	The Emotional Pie (Khalsa) Human Needs (Khalsa) Feelings Connection (Khalsa)
5 Coping Strategies	Handout of Coping Strategies (Robinson & Ward)
6 Relationships with Peers	Making Friends (Khalsa) Peer Pressure (Khalsa) Developing Constructive Romantic Relationships (Berman)
7 Family Relationships	Family Tree (Khalsa) Analyzing Parenting Behavior (Berman)
8 Changing Your Communications	Be Cool and Cool Off (Khalsa) Alternatives to Anger (Carrell) Changing My Communications (Khalsa) Changing Behaviors (Khalsa)

cus on change in order to avoid having the group become a "gripe session" for the girls. As the facilitator, it was important that I maintain enough emotional distance to control my own countertransference feelings, but not so much distance that I became disconnected from the girls or the group process. I traveled a considerable distance (40 miles each way) to facilitate the group, and at times it was difficult for me to accept the girls' attitudes. At these times, I would remind myself that their expressions of frustration were understandable, given their relational histories and current life situations, and that it was critical for them to have an opportunity to participate in a relationship where their authentic feelings and experiences could be heard and accepted. This perspective helped me maintain the necessary balance that allowed me to stay connected in spite of their efforts to distance themselves from me and the group experience.

Another external factor that influenced the therapeutic relationship was the emphasis within the facility on behavioral control. Although there was a treatment component within the milieu, it was essentially a correctional facility for delinquent girls. The need to control acting-out behaviors often led to power struggles between the staff and the girls, with the result being a "lock down" in the facility, wherein all privileges were suspended for some period of time. As stated earlier, it was mandatory that the girls participate in therapy, so girls rarely refused to attend the group. Nevertheless, the power struggles and control exercised by the staff often created a tense, negative atmosphere within the facility that spilled over into the group.

In order to address this area, I made a clear distinction between the group process and the milieu. I think that in some ways, it was helpful that I was not a regular member of the staff. The girls perceived me as an "outsider" who was helpful and was not involved in directly controlling their behavior. I could not independently give or take away points; therefore, during times of conflict, I was not perceived as an authority figure who was trying to have control over their lives. During the initial group sessions, I clarified my status and established boundaries for the group process, making it clear that we would not focus on the events that occurred within the milieu. For the most part, the girls respected this limit and it was possible to follow (with few exceptions) the planned curriculum for the group.

At other times, my auxiliary status within the facility was less desirable because it made it difficult to maintain effective, ongoing communication with the clinical staff. It was important for me to be aware of the climate in the residence each week as I entered to conduct the group, so that I had some preparation for what to expect from the girls. I was usually able to obtain this information, but it took time to develop the kind of relationships with the staff that facilitated these conversations. Despite these challenges, it was possible to successfully implement the group intervention, and to establish a context that allowed the girls to examine their relational skills.

MAJOR RELATIONAL THEMES AND CRITICAL JUNCTURES[1]

Three major relational themes emerged during the group: (1) feeling safe within relationships, (2) balancing the needs for self-respect and for survival, and (3) maintaining an authentic "self." Within each of these themes critical junctures occurred in the sessions, wherein the girls began

---

[1]All comments attributed to the girls are fictionalized composites derived from the types of comments that many of the girls made throughout the course of three different group cycles.

to examine their relational experiences and to think about ways that they could change their behavior. The first theme, safety in relationships, involved issues of physical, emotional, and psychological safety. Girls who had experienced abuse and/or neglect felt no sense of safety either at home or within the residential facility. They viewed all relationships (except those with a few close friends) as emotionally and/or physically dangerous. These girls tended to express extreme self-reliance and exhibited a marked distrust of others.

Meeting Safety Needs

For other girls, home had been a place of safety, and the residential facility was unsafe. In responding to an activity in which they were asked to describe situations associated with different feelings, these young women made statements such as "I feel accepted when my family supports me and believes in me"; "When I feel sad, I feel better when my mom gives me a hug; and "I will feel comfortable when I go home because I feel secure there." Being removed from their homes contributed to feelings of loss and insecurity for these girls, and their sole desire was to return home. While in the residential facility, girls were reluctant to develop meaningful relationships with staff or other residents, preferring to "do their time" and return to their home communities.

Although the theme of safety within relationships was a complicated one to address within the context of the residential facility, it was an important one to focus on in the group. This theme of safety was reflected in the process of developing trust within the group. The girls not only had difficulty trusting me (as the group facilitator), but they also had significant difficulty trusting each other. Learning to trust each other began with the establishment of ground rules for the group, which was done during the initial sessions. I was careful to introduce myself as the group facilitator to the girls in such a way that I conveyed a sense of mutuality and respect. The stance I took was one of authenticity and support. I consciously chose to disclose certain personal facts about my life when asked by the girls (e.g., that I am unmarried and have no children) in an effort to make myself more of a "real person" to them. I also gave supportive comments as the girls disclosed personal information about their own lives, in order to model the type of feedback that I was hoping to establish as the norm for the group. It was particularly important to strive to develop a therapeutic relationship in which all participants were seen, heard, and "known," to some extent. Because of their incarceration, the girls expected to have hierarchical, structured relationship with adults, who were perceived as authority figures with almost absolute power over their lives. I worked hard to present myself as a person who was approachable, interested in their well-being, and willing to be open about myself, while at the same time remaining aware of my position of power within the larger context of the residential facility.

The girls had experienced numerous betrayals of trust in their lives, and they were very articulate in the group discussions about their belief that few people could be trusted. This concern over trust led to the first critical juncture in the therapeutic relationship, which occurred during the fourth group session. During the initial three sessions they had cooperated with the group process and seemed to enjoy the activities and discussions. The girls completed activities that were designed to facilitate self-exploration and self-disclosure, and which gave them opportunities to give feedback to each other. They responded well to the activities, but they gave little, if any, feedback to each other. There seemed to be an unspoken understanding among the girls that it was permissible to talk about oneself, but not to comment on, or about, each other's experiences.

Throughout these initial sessions, the girls became more authentic in their communications with each other. However, their longstanding relational images contradicted this behavior and dictated the need to distance themselves from the group process in an effort to protect themselves from being hurt. As one young woman stated:

> "You can't trust anyone, especially other girls. They will knife you in the back. . . . It used to happen to me all of the time. So I learned not to trust other girls, or anyone, really. I just keep to myself, especially in this place . . . I mind my own business."

By the fourth session, the girls staged a mini "revolt" and expressed ambivalence about the group process, questioning its relevance to their lives. They seemed to be struggling to defend against feelings of vulnerability, and they used strategies of disconnection that were second nature for them. One girl's comment captures the sentiment of most of the group members:

> "This group is stupid! I don't have a problem with relationships!! My problem is being locked up in here. I don't see how talking about my feelings or myself can help me with *that* problem."

At this juncture, my feelings as the group facilitator were mixed. I was fully aware of the power I possessed in this context, as a result of the hierarchical nature of the relationships between "staff" and "residents" in a correctional facility. As noted, the facility used a behavioral management system in which the girls earned points for cooperating with program activities. I knew that their opposition and defiance could cause them to lose points, if I chose to take this stance. Yet dealing with the situation in this manner would have gone against the norm established in the early phase of the group to create mutually empowering, respectful relationships. Therefore, I chose to honor their strategies of disconnection and took the time in the group to work through their concerns about trust and confidentiality.

In processing the girls' feelings, it was important that I respond in ways that affirmed my commitment to open, authentic relationships in which each party's needs and wishes are heard and respected. It was a challenge to accept the girls' complaints, while at the same time supporting my position that the group's focus on self-understanding and relational skills could be helpful. An example of the dialogue that occurred in the group will help to make this process clearer:

PARTICIPANT 1: I don't understand why we have to talk about all of this stuff, since it won't make any difference when I get out of here. . . . I don't have any problems with my friends on the "out"; I only have problems getting along with these girls in here because they can't be trusted.

PARTICIPANT 2: All of these girls are just out to get you, if you know what I mean. . . . They don't care about you or anyone else.

PARTICIPANT 3: And I don't trust the staff in here either . . . And that includes you as well. How do I know what you will do with the information that I talk about in here? You could tell other people . . . my caseworker and stuff . . . and I'd be locked up even longer.

ELIZABETH: It sounds like trust is a real big issue for all of you. . . . Have there been times when the other girls and the staff have betrayed your trust?

PARTICIPANT 2: Plenty of times. . . . That's why I don't trust anyone in here. I just have to keep everything inside . . . I can't really talk about my feelings or what has happened to me.

PARTICIPANT 3: Well . . . some of the staff aren't so bad. . . . They have to keep things confidential—it's their job. But talking to staff isn't really going to help me. I've got to do this all myself—I have to make the changes that I need to make in order to stay out of trouble . . . no one can really help me with this—I have to do it all myself.

ELIZABETH: I can understand why you feel that you have to do everything yourself, given your experiences. But I'm hoping that the group can introduce you to another way to deal with this, perhaps help you begin to think about ways of being in relationships that don't involve your being betrayed or hurt. Hopefully, the group can help you think about the types of relationships you would like to have, and introduce you to some skills that might help you develop these sorts of relationships with important people in your life. I believe that by providing opportunities in the group for you to think about your relationships and the feelings that you have when you interact with others, it will be possible for you to learn more about yourselves and about relationships, and that new learning can help you get along better with others, both in here and outside, when you return to the community.

While acknowledging their feelings of discomfort with the group, I also affirmed my personal belief in the significance of the group and my desire to be helpful to them as they struggled to make sense of their lives and their incarceration. By the end of this group session, the girls and I were able to negotiate a "truce": We mutually agreed that those who felt that the group activities were not relevant or helpful could decline to participate. Since the facility mandated attendance at the group sessions, they would have to be present, but they agreed to sit quietly or read if they chose not to participate, and to not disrupt the group process. This agreement was upheld throughout the remaining group sessions. The girls came to each of the meetings, and if they chose not to participate in any of the activities, they quietly read or put their heads down on the desk. They often physically placed themselves outside of the group circle, but managed to stay connected to the group process in nonverbal (and sometimes verbal) ways.

This session was an important milestone for the group. My response to the "revolt" demonstrated my commitment to mutuality, empathy, and respect—the hallmarks of relational–cultural theory—in an overt way. The girls and I took the time to listen carefully to each other and to share our perspectives and feelings about the group process. I verbalized my understanding of their position, and I asked that they try to understand my position. In the end, we were able to gain something that was significant to each of us. The girls earned the right to refuse to participate in group activities without penalty, while I gained the right to conduct group sessions without being forced to manage disruptive behaviors. This session helped to create a group climate that facilitated increased authenticity over time, and led to a group experience that the girls reported as being helpful to their self-understanding and knowledge about the development and maintenance of positive relationships with others.

Working through the issues of safety and trust within the group was particularly challenging because of the girls' incarceration. Their forced separation from home and friends contributed to a longing to return home that often impaired their ability to remain aware of the reality of these relationships. It pushed any ambivalent feelings so far underground that only the more positive feelings were consciously experienced. This process was most poignantly seen when the focus of the sessions shifted to identifying positive relationships in their lives. The girls identified relationships with their mothers (and/or grandmothers) as the most important ones in their lives. As they talked in more detail about their relationships with maternal figures, they began to expose more of their authentic selves, which led to increased feelings of vulnerability. They acknowledged the disappointment they had caused their mothers and grandmothers by their delinquent behaviors, and the guilt they felt over behaving in ways in which their caretakers disapproved. The comments made by one of the girls represents the general sentiment that was expressed by most of the group members:

> "My mother is my best friend. I can trust her with anything . . . I tell her everything. She knows that some of the things I do are wrong, and she doesn't like it, but she sticks by me anyway. . . . I don't know what I would do if my mother ever died or anything. I know that I would want to die too—I just couldn't live without my mother. . . .
>
> "She was really angry with me . . . and disappointed when I got locked up. But she stuck by me anyway. . . . I feel bad for upsetting her like that, but I'm hoping that she will understand. . . ."

In one of the structured group exercises, the girls were asked to list their hopes and fears about the future. Many of their fears were relational in nature, such as the fear of losing their family, having a parent die, having their parents perceive them as failures, and being removed permanently from their families. These fears were particularly poignant because some of the girls had been separated from their families for 2 or more years, as they served time in different residential facilities. All expressed a hope that they would be successful and stay out of trouble, and many indicated that one of their highest hopes was to have a good relationship with their family members. Thus, as we moved through issues of safety and trust within the group, the girls were better able to get in touch with their longing for positive relationships with family members. They were also able to give and receive support from each other for their feelings, which provided an experience that challenged their relational images.

Balancing Self-Respect and Survival Needs

The second theme, that of balancing the need for self-respect with the need for survival, was experienced by the girls in both their home communities and within the facility. Most of the girls had histories of running away from home, whereupon they had been forced to rely on others for their survival. In these situations, the need to survive often compromised their sense of self-respect. At times, they were forced to become involved in personally distasteful and/or shameful experiences (e.g., prostitution and drug trafficking) in order to obtain basic necessities (such as food and shelter). During our group discussions, the girls struggled to make sense of these experiences. They knew that some of the behaviors in which they had engaged during a runaway incident were not reflective of their desires or wishes; however, they felt compelled to act in these ways in order to survive on the street.

Within the residential facility, the need to survive occurred on a different level. The girls were concerned with their emotional and psychological survival. They struggled to find ways of feeling good about themselves, while trying to cope with the uncertainty surrounding their follow-up placements. While incarcerated, the girls used such strategies as isolation and focusing on the here-and-now as ways of coping. They often felt a deep sense of loneliness but were reluctant to connect significantly with others inside the facility because of their need to survive the experience without being hurt. Some girls projected responsibility for their current feelings on the "system" (as represented by the residential staff). They focused almost exclusively on getting out of the facility and returning home. The girls seemed to make a commitment to maintain what they perceived to be a "safe" interpersonal distance from staff and the other residents in the facility by not engaging in relationships in which they revealed their authentic selves. As one young woman stated:

> "I just play the game while I'm in here. . . . I do what they want me to do, and that's all. I don't let anyone see the 'real me' like I do when I'm on the out. . . . "

These girls were engaging in strategies of disconnection in an effort to protect themselves from perceived harm.

Maintaining self-respect and surviving in the different environments wherein they find themselves is a complex issue for delinquent girls. Relational–cultural theory can help them make sense of this challenge. The need to survive is quite real for these young women, and not just in the physical and material ways that accompany a runaway incident. They also have a need to survive emotionally and psychologically in their relational lives, and often feel compelled to behave in ways that are not consistent with their self-identities. As we worked through this theme during the group sessions, the girls began to explore the complexities involved in their needs for self-respect and for survival. This process was seen most clearly in the sessions in which the girls were asked to make a commitment to the goal of personal change. The final three group sessions dealt with the girls' relationships with friends and family members. The activities were designed to help the girls get in touch with their feelings and explore their coping strategies. Almost all of the girls acknowledged problems with substance use/abuse and made the link between this behavior and their efforts to deal with their feelings. They reported feeling accepted by others when they used drugs, and angry with themselves when they were unable to control this use.

The link between their drug use and their affective states, and the tension associated with being accepted by peers versus controlling their drug use were issues that we revisited often in the group discussions. For many of the girls, their participation in drug use represented a central relational paradox. They had an intense desire to be accepted by their peers, so they used drugs. But they were also aware that this behavior caused them significant personal problems, including conflicts with their parents and the possibility of incarceration. In the past, many of the girls had altered their personal beliefs so that they would fit in with their friends who were using drugs. As we tried to work through the paradox in the group, the girls expressed a desire to become more authentic in these relationships, and to find ways to remain true to their convictions to remain drug-free following their release. They were able to acknowledge how difficult this would be, and we used the group discussions to explore how they might negotiate with their friends to refrain from using drugs, so that they would not need to terminate these relationships in order to remain drug-free.

As the focus of the group activities moved more deeply into the girls' relationships with their family members, it became clear that all had experienced situations in which they felt their needs had not been met by parental figures. The use of vignettes helped to facilitate this discussion and made it easier for the girls to explore their feelings toward their parents. As noted, these relationships were very important to the girls, and they felt disloyal and guilty when they described negative experiences with their parents in the group. The vignettes provided a sense of distance for the girls and enabled them to express their feelings of anger and frustration with a greater feeling of emotional safety. However, if their relationships with their parental figures are to become more authentic and mutual, it will be important for the girls to become better at articulating their needs to their parents and expressing when these needs are not being met.

Maintaining Authenticity

The third relational theme, that of maintaining authenticity within the context of significant relationships, was primarily seen in the girls' discussions of their relationships with boyfriends and close friends. Some of the girls held firm to their belief in the importance of always being true to self within these relationships, whereas others felt that they could not be authentic because of the fear of rejection. They were aware of feeling the tension between being accepted by others and being true to self, but they were unable to identify ways to resolve it. For many of the girls, the "price" for authenticity in relationships was felt to be too high—it meant being rejected and/or abandoned. Relational–cultural theory explains this dilemma as a consequence of the girls' experiences of disconnection in relationships. The theory also provides guidelines that therapists can use to facilitate change. Using the tenets of the theory, I was able to explain to the girls that their need to remain in connection was so important that they were willing to change aspects of themselves in order to better "fit" the expectations of others. The girls slowly learned to identify the relational binds in which they often found themselves, and they were introduced to ways of attempting to renegotiate these relationships once they returned to their home communities.

Relational–cultural theory calls for the development of relationships that are mutually empowering, in the sense that the emotional and relational needs of those involved are responded to and validated. The girls desperately wanted to improve their relationships with their parents, particularly with their mothers, and hoped to behave differently when they were released from the facility. Relational–cultural theory also tells us that for relationships to be mutual, it is necessary for *both* individuals to change. The girls continued to hold an individualistic orientation and resisted the perspective highlighted in relational–cultural theory, that growth and healthy psychological/emotional development occur *in relationship* with others. Despite my efforts to convey the importance of working together with others to make the changes for which they hoped, as well as the need for ongoing therapy for both the girls and their parents if these relationships were going to change for the better, the girls held firm to their beliefs. As we moved into a discussion of the change process in the final session, the girls were convinced that they could make the necessary changes in their own behavior to improve relationships with significant people in their lives. They were unable to identify the supportive resources they would need to implement and sustain the changes they hoped to make following discharge. They were convinced that they alone could do whatever was necessary to change their negative relationships without the active participation of their parents or friends. The girls vacillated between feeling positive about their own ability to make changes, and feeling fearful that they might succumb to the old pressures and resume old behaviors (e.g., drug use and running away from home).

There were times during these final group sessions when I became discouraged and frustrated. The statistics on recidivism in female delinquents indicate that about 70% ends up returning to delinquent behaviors; these girls are reincarcerated within 1 year of their release from a residential facility. I realized that the girls' needs for relational connections were so strong that they would have tremendous difficulty removing themselves from situations where their friends were involved in behaviors that they knew could lead to their arrest and reincarceration. They would also have difficulty altering the relational and communication patterns between themselves and their parental figures. The girls were still somewhat resistant to therapy, and I knew that the problems in their relational lives would not change without ongoing therapeutic intervention. I had to work hard to hold onto the recognition that the therapeutic relationship I had developed with the group was only one step in a long process of change for these girls. I used the final session to point out the positive changes that the girls had made as a result of their involvement in the therapeutic program at the facility, reinforced the insights they had developed as a result of the group sessions, and reminded them of the support they had both given to, and received from, others over the 8-week period.

CONCLUSIONS AND TREATMENT RECOMMENDATIONS

Incarcerated delinquent girls are a challenging population with which to work therapeutically. Yet they are in desperate need of effective, gender-specific treatment approaches designed to address their multiple needs. The relational lives of these young women are complex and more often than not reflect repeated disconnections and disruptions in significant, primary relationships. The girls have learned various strategies of protecting themselves within relationships; these strategies generally leave them feeling sad, isolated and angry. By the time they are incarcerated, they typically have experienced a series of relationships wherein they have been betrayed, hurt, and disappointed. Trust, understandably, is a central issue for this population. And yet, these girls have not avoided connecting with others. The need to remain in connection with others is equally as strong as the fear of rejection, and so they manage to build relationships in whatever ways they can. Some of these connections are positive, in the sense that the girls manage to get at least some of their needs met within the relationship. Others are more detrimental to the girls' development, particularly when they feel compelled to alter significant parts of themselves in an effort to maintain these relationships. The group intervention described in this case study attempted to address this area of the girls' lives, and it used the tenets of relational–cultural theory to develop and guide the therapeutic process.

At the end of the group experience I was left with many questions about the extent to which the girls had experienced a mutually empathic therapeutic relationship within the group. The feedback that I received from the staff made it clear that the girls often spoke about missing my presence in the facility and had very positive things to say about the group experience to their caseworkers and attorneys during case conferences. This information was encouraging and has helped to sustain my commitment to the importance of providing this type of a group intervention for incarcerated delinquent girls.

It can be challenging to establish a mutual, authentic, therapeutic relationship within the context of a correctional facility. In spite of the challenges posed by the institutional environment, however, it is possible for a therapist to develop such relationships by exhibiting patience, understanding, and authenticity. Correctional facilities for delinquents are hierarchical in structure, and staff focus primarily on maintaining behavioral control within the institution. In order to facilitate growth-enhancing relationships between staff and residents in these facilities, it would be important that *all* staff (clinical, milieu, and administrative) work in collaboration to establish interactions that are respectful, authentic, and trustworthy. Doing so would require a consensus among the staff in the facility that developing positive, growth-enhancing relationships with the girls and among themselves is a priority that warrants time, attention, specific training, and structural supports. Once this perspective becomes firmly established within a facility, it shapes the ways in which staff and residents interact and reinforces the clinical focus on growth-fostering relationships.

The group intervention described in this case study was conducted in relative isolation, in the sense that there was no formal involvement of nonclinical staff in the process. The milieu and administrative staff were aware of the group's existence but had very little information about its content or focus. Thus they were not able to work in collaboration with the clinical staff, to reinforce the perspective on relationships being presented in the group, during their everyday interactions with the girls. This noninvolvement was a limitation of the intervention and one that I hope will receive greater attention as we continue to implement the group at this facility. Ideally, all staff should receive training in relational–cultural theory and work in conjunction with the group facilitators to develop mutually empathic, authentic relationships with the residents.

It would also be helpful to provide at least some opportunity for residents to participate in self-governing activities (such as a peer council that could handle minor conflicts between girls). Through these sorts of activities, girls could be helped to engage in positive, growth-enhancing relationships with staff and each other; such experiences could provide a sort of *in vivo* experience of the perspective and information presented in the group. Altering the general attitude within juvenile correctional facilities from a focus on behavioral control to one of establishing therapeutic, positive relationships with young people is a challenge. The good news is that the field of juvenile justice is slowly moving in that direction. Relational-cultural theory can provide a theoretical framework to guide this work and should be given careful consideration in the development of gender-specific treatments for delinquent girls.

REFERENCES

Belknap, J., Dunn, M., & Holsinger, K. (1997). *Moving toward juvenile justice and youth-serving systems that address the distinct experience of the adolescent female.* Report to the Governor, Office of Criminal Justice Services, Columbus, OH.

Berman, P. (1994). *Therapeutic exercises for victimized and neglected girls: Applications for individual, family and group psychotherapy.* Sarasota, FL: Professional Resource Press.

Bowers, L., & Klein, W. (1983). The etiology of female juvenile delinquency and gang membership: A test of psychological and social structural explanations. *Adolescence, 18,* 739–751.

Carrell, S. (1993). *Group exercises for adolescents: A manual for therapists.* Newbury Park, CA: Sage.

Chesney-Lind, M. (1987). Girls and violence: An exploration of the gender gap in serious delinquent behavior. In D. H. Crowell, I. M. Evens, & C. R. O'Donnell (Eds.), *Childhood aggression and violence: Sources of influence, prevention and control* (pp. 87–131). New York: Plenum Press.

Chesney-Lind, M. (1997). *The female offender: Girls, women, and crime.* Thousand Oaks, CA: Sage.

Fejes-Mendoza, K., Miller, D., & Eppler, R. (1995). Portraits of dysfunction: Criminal, educational, and family profiles of juvenile female offenders. *Education and Treatment of Children, 18*(3), 309–321.

Ginsberg, C. (1981). Who are the women in prison? *American Correctional Association Monographs Series, 1*(1), 51–56.

Jordan, J. V. (1986). The meaning of mutuality. *Work in Progress, No. 23.* Wellesley, MA: Stone Center Working Paper Series.

Jordan, J. V., Kaplan, A. G., Miller, J. B., Stiver, I. P., & Surrey, J. I. (Eds.). (1991). *Women's growth in connection: Writings from the Stone Center.* New York: Guilford Press.

Khalsa, S. S. (1996). Group exercises for enhancing social skills and self-esteem. Sarasota, FL: Professional Resource Press.

Miller, J. B. (1988). Connections, disconnections, and violations. *Work in Progress, No. 33.* Wellesley, MA: Stone Center Working Paper Series.

Miller, J. B., Jordan, J. V., Kaplan, A. G., Stiver, I. P., & Surrey, J. (1991). Some misconceptions and reconceptions of a relational approach. *Work in Progress, No. 49.* Wellesley, MA: Stone Center Working Paper Series.

Miller, J. B., & Stiver, I. P. (1997). *The healing connection: How women form relationships in therapy and life.* Boston: Beacon Press.

Pipher, M. (1994). *Reviving Ophelia: Saving the selves of adolescent girls.* New York: Ballantine Books.

Robinson, T., & Ward, J. V. (1991). A belief far greater than anyone's unbelief: Cultivating resistance among African American female adolescents. In C. Gilligan, A. G. Rogers, & D. L. Tolman (Eds.), *Women, girls and psychotherapy: Reframing resistance* (pp. 87–103). New York: Haworth Press.

Index